ATTENTION DEFICIT DISORDER IN ADULTS

ATTENTION DEFICIT DISORDER IN ADULTS

A Different Way of Thinking

Fourth Edition

Lynn Weiss, Ph.D.

TAYLOR TRADE PUBLISHING

Lanham • New York • Dallas • Boulder • Toronto • Oxford

First Taylor Trade Publishing edition 2005

This Taylor Trade Publishing paperback edition of *Attention Deficit Disorder in Adults, Fourth Edition* is an original publication. It is published by arrangement with the author.

Published by Taylor Trade Publishing
An imprint of The Rowman & Littlefield Publishing Group, Inc.
4501 Forbes Boulevard, Suite 200
Lanham, Maryland 20706

Distributed by National Book Network

Library of Congress Cataloging-in-Publication Data

Weiss, Lynn.
Attention deficit disorder in adults : a different way of thinking / Lynn Weiss.— 4th ed.
p. cm.
"First Taylor Trade Publishing edition 2005."
ISBN 1-58979-237-8 (pbk. : alk. paper)
1. Attention-deficit disorder in adults—Popular works. I. Title.
RC394.A85W445 2005
616.85'89—dc22 2005004657

∞™ The paper used in this publication meets the minimum requirements of American National Standard for Information Sciences—Permanence of Paper for Printed Library Materials, ANSI/NISO Z39.48-1992.
Manufactured in the United States of America.

I dedicate this book to all people regardless of their brainstyle. May those of us who feel as if something is wrong with us know the truth, which is that each of us is wonderful and needed as we are made. May we know that one brainstyle is not superior or more normal than another. And may those who label and judge one brainstyle as acceptable and others as pathological come to know the truth that a broader perspective brings. May we work together to make the world a better place in which to live because of an acceptance of another aspect of human diversity. The world will truly become a better place as a result.

CONTENTS

ACKNOWLEDGMENTS

Special thanks to all the people over the years who have taught me through love, friendship, mentorship, and aggravation to understand diversity more fully in all of its forms.

The working team that has joined me in the production of this fourth edition deserves not only a vote of thanks, but also applause for a job well done. Let me begin by acknowledging Cat Long, a friend and artistic comrade who assisted me with inspiration and friendship during the years of my work with Attention Deficit Disorder. She tangled with some of the details that threatened to swamp me. Then there's Fleeta Cunningham and Tiffany Green, Bastrop Writers' Group stalwarts who have walked with me emotionally during this rewrite.

Camille Cline, my not-so-old old editor, has filled a niche that my brainstyle tends to leave blank. Her linear propensities coupled with her willingness to meet me halfway have allowed me to bring this project to a higher level than I could have accomplished alone. And appreciation to Janet Harris, who helped complete the editing, along with the Taylor production staff whom I haven't met, but greatly appreciate.

Keith Caramelli, M.D., and Al Galves, Ph.D., each brought his special expertise to bear in covering bases I could not reach—in medication and expanding approaches to the direction that I believe ADD must go.

And finally, to my special colleague and friend, John Rubel, Psy.D. I not only give thanks to him, but also wish to say that without his intellectual and emotional support, this edition might not have happened. He walked by my side as I struggled for several years to find a way to get my particular ADD perspective into words that would have a chance to raise the consciousness of readers to a new level. His moral support, caring, and teamwork made all this possible. Thank you, John.

TWENTY-NINE POSITIVE ATTRIBUTES OF ADD

1. Sensitive
2. Empathetic with the feelings of others
3. Feels things deeply
4. Creative in nature (including problem solving)
5. Inventive
6. Often sees things from a unique perspective
7. Great at finding things that are lost
8. Perceptually acute
9. Stand-up comic
10. Spontaneous
11. Fun
12. Energetic
13. Open and unsecretive
14. Eager for acceptance and willing to work for it
15. Responsive to positive reinforcement
16. Doesn't harbor resentment
17. Quick to do what one likes to do
18. Difficult to fool

19. Looks past surface appearance to the core of people, situations, and issues
20. Down to earth
21. Good networker
22. Sees unique relationships between people and things
23. Cross-disciplinary and interdisciplinary
24. Less likely to get in a rut or go stale
25. Original, with a sense of humor
26. Observant
27. Loyal
28. Intense when interested in something
29. More likely to do things because they want to than because they *should*, thus often wholehearted in efforts

FOREWORD

John G. Rubel

It helps to name something in order to talk about it. My guess is that you picked up this book because the term Attention Deficit Disorder (ADD)* has some relevance to your life. Perhaps a health-care professional diagnosed you with ADD, or through self-assessment you labeled yourself, or you know someone with ADD. But what does it mean to be ADD?

Psychologist George Kelly, the father of personal construct theory, believed it was important to first understand the labeler's frame of reference before looking at the individual being labeled. The majority of Western health-care professionals and educators, that is, the official labelers, believe that given a highly structured, cognitively driven academic curriculum, children should be able to focus their attention and control their behavior in order to maximize their learning potential.

Inherent in this belief is a value judgment. Children whose brainstyles may better fit a more active, experiential, applied,

* ADD and ADHD are used synonymously for the purposes of this book.

creative curriculum are frequently labeled ADD—a label that rips at the fabric of their human essence.

Another implicit value judgment in the ADD label is the notion of dyscontrol. An ADD diagnosis implies a person experiences inadequate control over and impairment of feelings, thoughts, and behaviors over which a "normal" person is believed to have adequate control. No society can survive without establishing its criteria for normalcy. However, societal value judgments reflecting a consensus based on an exhaustive dialogue among all community members tend to be the most reliable and valid.

It's doubtful that this is the manner in which ADD was determined to be a mental disorder, especially since the major community participants were selected mental health professionals and pharmaceutical companies, both of whom have high stakes in the outcome.

Philosopher Friedrich Nietzsche stated, "There are no facts, only interpretations." In the new and extensively revised edition of *Attention Deficit Disorder in Adults*, Dr. Lynn Weiss explores the many facets of individuals who have an ADD neurobiological brainstyle and offers practical, effective strategies to help people maximize their inherent capabilities. Readers will better understand the diversity of brainstyle construction, resulting in greater freedom to choose to be who they are or to modify their natural brainstyle to fit the normalcy of their culture.

First and foremost, this book should be read by anyone labeled ADD. I hesitate to use the word *should*, but Weiss's professional insights, applied knowledge, compassion, and sensitivity make this a luminous book that will validate and brighten the self-worth of individuals with an ADD brainstyle. This book was designed taking into account how ADD brainstyles process written material, so it will be easier and more enjoyable to read.

Family members, friends, and coworkers of individuals with an ADD brainstyle will also derive significant benefits from this book. They will better understand how an ADD brainstyle impacts relationships. Most importantly, they will learn how to validate, support, and encourage the people they care about whose brainstyles may be different.

Health-care professionals and educators working with adults who have an ADD brainstyle will find this book a refreshing and valuable resource. Weiss's clinical insights and practical suggestions are the culmination of over 40 years of professional and personal experience with this adult population. Her integration of brainstyle diversity theory, applied research, and clinical practice will enhance professionals' understanding of ADD brainstyles and lead to more effective, comprehensive interventions.

As a corollary to Nietzsche's quote, I say, "Choose your interpretations wisely." Reading *Attention Deficit Disorder in Adults* is a wise choice.

John S. Rubel, Psy.D., ABPP
Diplomate in Clinical Psychology
American Board of Professional Psychology

A NOTE FROM THE AUTHOR

One day, an epiphany came crashing in upon me. The awareness changed my life and, subsequently, the lives of many others. I realized why school had been so painful for me, so hard, unrewarding, and demoralizing. Insight flooded through me as I gained an answer for the feelings of inadequacy and low self-esteem I'd borne for years.

A doctor of philosophy degree and years of considerable success as a professional mental health clinician had failed to diminish the hard-core sense that something was amiss—something was *wrong* with me.

At the same time, however, I knew and had always known a different reality about myself. In contrast to the feelings of inadequacy, this perspective carried a feeling of inner wonder, creativity, and wisdom. In one way, I totally trusted my unique observations and insights, though they went unsupported by my teachers and, later, my colleagues. I didn't fit the cultural definition of smartness. My understanding and perspectives were simply not shared by the intellectual powers. Yet I believed in them without doubt.

Until my son ran into the barrier created by linear learning requirements and a belief system that shaped the educational environment in which he found himself, I had not seen a way to resolve the opposites that existed within myself. Suddenly, a resolution appeared—one that fit for both my son and myself, and as it turns out, for many, many other people.

I, too, with a brain construction like my son's, had trudged and fought my way through school and, later, the job market. Because I could do an adequate job and was an oversocialized, overly conscientious female, I had survived. But I lost my life. I would now say, "I lost touch with my True Self."

With the new insight, it was as if a huge weight fell away from my body, and I regained myself. All because I suddenly saw that my ability to perform and feel good about how I am is directly related to:

- the fit between my style of brain construction and the style in which I am being taught,
- the ways in which I am allowed to accomplish my goals, and
- the way in which I am evaluated.

I realized that my success, as well as those of others, cannot be measured by my "success" in the world when that is measured by the *way* in which we are made to accomplish our goals, if that way does not fit our neurobiological brainstyle. Our style of brain construction, measured against an artificially applied standard by an outside judge, does not provide an objective standard for our proficiency. One size or style does not fit all.

As I found ways to help my son survive and develop his True Self, I also gave permission for myself to do things in ways that fit me. Though gravely wounded as a child and young adult, I came to the *belief* that there never had been anything *wrong* with me; nor was there anything *wrong* with my son. Instead, I realized we each had our ways of thinking, perceiving, and doing that are shared by many others and are different from the ways of many others. I blossomed, and my work carried a message that others like me could use to release them from the prisons of their minds—prisons created by a psychosocial belief.

Before I fully understood the basis for the trauma that had hurt me, I underwent several years of psychotherapy. As I learned about the ADD facet of my wounding, I rethought what I'd learned earlier and did further healing of the Wounded Me. I spent much time journaling and studying my reactions to what I felt and the way in which I reacted to everyday events. But it was my work with my son and the many people who came to me over the years that aided my healing the most. Through them, I often saw my own journey portrayed. And through the creative solutions to their healing I saw solutions for my own ADD-related wounding.

When the groups first began to gather at my Dallas office in the mid-'80s, I came to know the nonclinical ways for healing and training those of us with an ADD brainstyle. The Accommodating Me gained skills to build the bridges back to the True Me so that I could become truly whole.

It was with this background that I retired from private practice and city life to a small town in central Texas to write about what

I'd learned. In the ten years since that change, I've accomplished two major things in relation to Attention Deficit Disorder. First, I've studied, through observation and introspection, how people learn, create, and express. And I've become increasingly aware of the many pathways to success that are available for each of us who allows herself purposely or unconsciously to find and live her fit.

Second, and perhaps of even greater consequence, I've discovered that the way to feel good about ourselves is to be who we naturally are rather than trying to mend or morph into a psychosocial or academic standard that doesn't fit. Not only have I purposely benefited from this discovery, but I also recognize that passing this legacy to my children, grandchildren, and their children, ad infinitum, will make the world a better place to live.

Thus, given the opportunity to update *Attention Deficit Disorder in Adults*, I jumped at the chance to share what I've learned in a life that spans seven decades. It's a good way to celebrate.

INTRODUCTION

I can only hope and pray that never again will a child be born who, at any point in his or her life, is given a label that in any way will diminish his or her unique wonderfulness—the wonderfulness of diversity, regardless of style of brain construction.

I now know this is what I wish for. I did not know it when I first became personally aware of what is labeled Attention Deficit Disorder (ADD) or Attention Deficit Hyperactivity Disorder (ADHD). I will use the term ADD throughout this work to include both ADD and ADHD.

Now I know that Attention Deficit Disorder does not need to be the devastating condition that it was previously thought to be. Having it certainly doesn't mean you have a mental condition or are disordered. You will appear to be disabled, however, *if you're placed in situations that do not fit your brainstyle.*

In this book, I plan to address the pain, suffering, and everyday problems that afflict you by being repeatedly placed in situations that don't fit your brainstyle—problems that result from a lack of understanding on your part. I will also address this lack of understanding as simply an issue of ignoring ADD as a human diversity issue. And, finally, I will address a judgment-free True You who has talents and skills that are not only valuable but that are also needed to bring wholeness and health to the world.

MY PERSONAL ADD STORY

Let me start my personal story by sharing how I got into this whole ADD thing in the first place. I certainly didn't plan it, nor did I have any idea during my clinical training in the 1960s that I would end up spending years of my professional career deeply embedded in ADD work.

It all started when my son's fourth-grade teacher told me, "He could do his work, if he'd just settle down." I began to realize that a thing called Attention Deficit Disorder was present in my family. I didn't do much about it then. I didn't know *what* to do. Besides, I thought, as most psychotherapists and mental health professionals did at the time, that it would disappear when my son reached puberty.

It wasn't until he was thirteen that my eyes were opened and I understood that ADD was a lifelong condition. My son's inability to block out the high level of activity in junior high caused him to become a frequent visitor to the principal's office. And he began to do poorly in math, the subject in which he had always excelled, because he couldn't concentrate on all the steps involved. He would make careless errors even when he understood the concepts.

I had him thoroughly evaluated for ADD and discovered he wasn't outgrowing it. In fact, far from disappearing, as we had expected it to, it was causing him more trouble than before. And during the course of my son's evaluation, his father, by then my ex-husband, was evaluated as being ADD, too.

It was then that I realized how ADD shapes personality, torments its *victims*, and fragments relationships. I did not yet realize that there were many positive ADD attributes or that many of the problems caused by ADD could be avoided by training a child to accommodate to a linear world that doesn't fit, but in which a person can learn to function. These insights came several years later.

At about the same time that I learned about my son and his father, I had two adult clinical psychotherapy patients who were not responding to treatment, and I noticed they had attentional problems similar to those present in schoolchildren. When I went to the professional literature hoping to find alternative treatment for them, I discovered an article entitled, "The Diagnosis and Treatment of Attention Deficit Disorder, Residual Type," by David Woods, in *Psychiatric Annals* 16, no. 1 (January 1986) that outlined the condition in adults.

Then, on my radio talk show at KLIF in Dallas, I mentioned ADD in adults and its characteristics. I watched as the phone lines lit up instantly and the switchboard accumulated a record number of requests for further information. I soon found myself deluged with requests for information about ADD in adults.

But I had very little information to offer. In my research I'd discovered there was precious little available, and what was available was scientifically oriented and not helpful to the general public. As a result, I did what my clinical training had taught me to do. I developed screening procedures, seminars, workshops, and group educational/counseling sessions.

An analogy of sending a fish to flying school made its way into my talks and workshops. The fish's inability to fly in no way indicates that it cannot successfully procure food, develop skills for successful transportation, or develop its potential to live a successful, happy life. The fish analogy slowly led me to my way of viewing ADD—a way that has taken over my present thinking about ADD and has led me to what people with ADD attributes need to do in order to have the opportunity to become fully functioning adults in all aspects of life.

MY EARLY OBSERVATIONS OF ADD

Initially, my work with ADD was called "Treatment of ADD" because that is the perspective I learned in school. I began, however, to see that there are as many positive ADD attributes as negative ones. After I realized this, I went through a period when I called what I did "Training in the use of the ADD way of living." Next, I realized that people with a predominantly linear brainstyle have as many problems as those of us who demonstrate ADD attributes.

The epiphany that crashed into my conscious awareness in 1996 was that the problems we have, regardless of whether we have an ADD or linear brainstyle, occur when there is a lack of fit between our brainstyle and the kind of work we are attempting to accomplish.

If you have many ADD characteristics, then you will have trouble with tasks that are linear in nature, such as those that require close attention to detail. However, if you have many linear attributes, then you will have trouble with tasks that are nonlinear, such as seeing the overall patterns inherent in a task before you see the details. I was able to verify that linear people develop the same symptoms of inattentiveness, reactivity, impulsivity, lack of follow-through, and so on when they are expected to function in a nonlinear ADD-style environment.

To effectively utilize your style of brain to accomplish tasks, to learn, achieve, and demonstrate what you know that fits your brainstyle, you must be able to work using the style inherent in your brain's construction. This is true for everyone, not just for people with many ADD attributes. Also, tests of everyone's level of achievement must utilize testing methods that fit a person's brainstyle. The goals stay the same. The testing methods change.

These steps have led me to a synthesis of my insights that outlines a three-pronged approach to dealing with ADD. Actually, this same three-pronged approach works for linear people, but I choose to focus on its significance for ADD at this time. These I pass on to you, whether you have a lot of ADD attributes or a few.

A THREE-PRONGED PERSPECTIVE ON ADD

Prong 1: The True You

First and foremost, it is *essential* to understand that there is nothing inherently *wrong* or *disordered* with you as a person who has a few, some, or many ADD attributes. You have a natural style of brain construction—one with which you are born. I call this the True You. It is from the core of your True Self that your talents and skills grow. Or, if your True Self lay dormant or has been disallowed, it will be the skills and talents that come into full bloom as originally intended from your True Self.

Your True You is the unwarped, unjudged, unwounded, natural you. All of the original innate skills, talents, attributes, and gifts with which you were born are available to you to use as you choose. And they can lead you to accomplish any goal you desire by following pathways to learning and achievement that reflect the way in which your True You does business.

Unfortunately, if you have ADD characteristics, the True Self rarely had the opportunity to flourish in a supportive environment that allowed you to approximate your potential. As a result, you became wounded. You likely lost self-esteem and confidence in yourself. You became separated from using and enjoying the way in which you were made. You undoubtedly bumped into situations that did not fit your natural style of learning and working. You most likely felt bruised. As a result, you also probably learned to disregard your natural resources for learning and accomplishing things so that they went underground, out of your conscious awareness.

Prong 2: The Wounded You

The result of your experience is that you have been hurt, though probably unintentionally. You must learn how you can heal those hurts so you can effectively reconnect with the True You. You must become aware of the right environment to support your brainstyle—one that serves the needs of your True Self—so you can retrieve your lost skills and talents.

In today's world, there are three typical causes of injury that you are likely to have suffered:

- Socialization—All societies have beliefs about what are proper ways for their members to behave. When these beliefs do not reflect the reality and diversity of how humans are made, wounding results. If, for example, sitting still in school is thought to indicate a high level of socialization, then those of us who learn by being active will be hurt. It's that simple.

- The Learning of Harmful Beliefs—Wounding happens when a person believes there is only one acceptable way to be, to do, to think, or to live. All other ways, the result of different innate skills and talents, are considered flawed. Previously, beliefs have been the business of religion, but the damage done by beliefs has now spread through medicine, education, employment, and the legal system.

  Labeling ADD/ADHD as a disability and placing it within the Americans with Disabilities Act is an example of such a belief.

- The Leveling of Judgments—If a person with the untapped resources of the True Self is judged to be pathological because his or her natural way of doing things doesn't fit the current social model, the person is wounded by virtue of being judged. This applies to people labeled with ADD. They are even said to have a medical problem, are often denied an education that fits their brain construction, and are judged for work by standards that preclude their showing what they can do.

If you are in this situation, you are not only thwarted from using your natural talents but you must also be labeled *disabled* in order to be given an opportunity to achieve. Further damage comes from having to admit publicly, "There is something *wrong* with me. That's why I'm being given accommodation."

Secondary Wounding. Further damage occurs when you have bought into the belief that your innate way is wrong. Self-depreciation results, and it continues damaging you as long as the belief persists.

If you are required to do something that doesn't fit who you are, and you resist, complain, react, or become depressed, anxious, clumsy, or indecisive, you are likely to be scolded, chastised, or further labeled because you've reacted. When you resist, you are likely to be called oppositional. When you complain, you may be called argumentative. When you cry or become depressed, you are called symptomatic. When you become anxious, you are given a pathological label and medication to deal with your anxiety.

But these secondary symptoms are only the result of being pressured or forced to do something that doesn't fit you in the first place—something that is out of alignment with what is in the best interest of the True You. Then when you are additionally labeled with behavioral or emotional problems, you are wounded a second time.

This latter wounding of you does not need to happen. The secondary problems or symptoms are not inherently a part of the original True Self. The behaviors and feelings are only indicators that something is amiss with the relationship between your way and the environment in which you are living. Instead of your needing to change, the environment may need to be changed. The True You needs to be saved from being required to do what doesn't fit. When that happens, the secondary symptoms disappear.

Prong 3: The Accommodating You

Even when you have rediscovered the True You and know the kinds of settings in which you can optimally function, you will encounter the imperfect world of everyday life. Living in this imperfect world means you will not always be able to find a fit between your natural ways and the environments you face. But you can learn skills to bridge the differences between your innate skills and the expectations placed on you. And you can do this without hurting yourself further.

As you become aware of the True You, you will learn to recognize how well your surroundings fit you. You'll become attuned to beliefs that honor you. Simultaneously, you will continue to respond the best you can until you can do something to make the changes you need.

On a personal level, you will be able to make plans, aligning your everyday life with the needs of the True You. But such moves take time. Take, for example, a move to self-employment. This will require time to adjust your finances, family obligations, and inner courage before you can actually make the step. You may also need to acquire some new skills. While you are acquiring the tools you need to make such moves, you will learn to accommodate your current situation so you are not further wounded.

Always remember, you are perfect the way you are naturally constructed. Know that your untapped resources are desperately needed not only by you but also by the society in which you live. But also know that there is usually a considerable lag between any new way to look at a situation and the actual changing of society to accommodate that new perspective.

All three of these prongs may need to be implemented if you are to reach your full potential. As you heal and accommodate, you must believe that there is nothing inherently *wrong* with you because you have an ADD style of brain construction. This is a fundamental position you must take. You deserve it.

It may mean you have to resist what others think or say about you. Authorities may tell you differently. Words may lead you to think you are inferior, for labels wound you as surely as fists. The very words, Attention Deficit Disorder, associated with your style of brain construction carry a damaging message. But you can pull courage from within yourself to simply refuse to accept what is cast your way. You can reach out to those of us who are not afraid of brainstyle diversity. You can use us as models as you safeguard the True You while healing the Wounded You and as you entice an imperfect world with the Accommodating You. That is what this book is about.

What I recall in my personal story is the heart-wrenching, gut-tightening reaction I felt upon hearing my son labeled. My mind feared that my wonderful child would not be able to "make it" in life. He was, after all, *disordered.*

"Not my son," I screamed silently. "Not this resourceful child who in our home keeps up fine with our high-functioning family and who also did so well in preschool."

His ability to function—to create, problem solve, invent, and relate expressively to others, children and adults alike—was in good working order until he was pressed into a desk and required to learn what someone else thought he ought to learn in a certain time and ways they thought he ought to learn it. Suddenly, he developed problems and became deficient.

To save my son, I quickly began to spend hours at school brokering the system on his behalf. I found teachers and counselors who didn't shame and punish him. And I learned to restrict the time he was allowed to spend doing work at home—the same work he couldn't manage at school. I changed the way he was being taught to one that fit the way he learned, and he learned adequately—not up to potential, but adequately.

And by seventh grade, I placed him on medication to assist him in managing his ADD. At the end of the year, he won the citizenship award for most improved behavior. He passed pre-algebra, too.

In retrospect, I feel sad that I had to turn to medication to get him through a situation that didn't fit him. Yet I understand now, as I did at the time, that without it, he was in more risk of being damaged. It was a treatment that helped him survive an ill-fitting environment.

My hope is that this book will add to the steps being taken so children do not need to be medicated in order to survive a learning environment that is inappropriate for their style of brain construction. For this to happen, we parents and other adults must educate ourselves to what we can do about the natural diversity of our brainstyles. And we must gather our courage and become spokespersons to advocate for fair treatment for all, regardless of the style of the True Selves. Then all people can work together for everyone's best outcome.

LIFE WITH ADD: REAL PEOPLE'S STORIES

LASHAWNA'S STORY: EMBRACING AN ADD DIAGNOSIS

Are you expected to do a job that you weren't hired to do and that you can't do? That's what happened to LaShawna.

I was hired to file and make copies. I don't like sitting behind a desk and I'm not good with details, so it was a good job for me. Well, the next thing I know, they go and change me to another job. I hate change. It takes me a long time to get used to new things—there's always so much to learn when everything is new.

Now I have to sit at the switchboard all day. And when I'm not taking calls I'm supposed to be doing paperwork—whatever anyone wants to give me. It's never the same from one moment to the next.

I'm real sensitive, too. And people just throw things on the desk. They're not nice to me. They tell me I don't do things fast enough. Don't they know I'm totally confused by all this changing? They are mean to me. They hurt my feelings.

Worst of all, I'm afraid I'll lose my job even though I hate it. But I have to keep it because I always lose jobs that I get.

SAM'S STORY: TAKING A LITTLE OF THIS AND THAT

Do you feel that you never again want to go anywhere near school even though you worry that if you don't, maybe you won't be able to make a living doing what you'd like to do? That's what happened to Sam.

Man, I remember how awful school was when I was a kid. Everyone was trying to help me—but I didn't want help. I wanted out of school.

I felt like a real loser. Maybe I still am. My brother and folks are all smart, but I never could make the grades. I could barely stand to sit all day in school, but then I was expected to go home and do more sitting to get my homework done. I could sit down to play my guitar, but people just said that was because I wanted to play my guitar. So it was bad that I didn't sit in school and bad that I did sit playing my guitar. Boy, no matter what I did, I couldn't win.

I put my foot down, finally. I played my guitar anyway and fished a lot. I liked that, too. But I guess playing a 12-string guitar and fishing and knowing about everything there is to know about the fish in the gulf must be easy if I could do it.

I used to see my mom crying because she thought I'd never be able to make a living. Well I'm not smart, but I'm not stupid, either. I'll do something—I hope.

ALISHA'S STORY: ON-AGAIN, OFF-AGAIN ADD

Do you have plenty of intelligence, education, work experience, and talents, but discover you have run up against an obstacle that could block your reaching your dream—a dream you are capable of performing but one that requires more training in a form you can't achieve?

The first eight years of my life were spent on a riverboat. The crew and my parents taught me everything I needed to know. But my life took a turn for the worse when I was put ashore and confined to a school desk for long hours. I felt caged. My aptitude test scores were high, but I sure couldn't keep up with all those little dinky tests and homework papers.

I got through school despite failing to live up to my potential and found I was happier when I was working as a teacher, coach, and counselor. My life was pretty much working for me, that is, until the dream to become a minister hit me. I became dedicated to the heartfelt idea of helping people in this new way. I envisioned the type of ministry I would have. Wow!

But suddenly I find myself back in the cage with constant assignments that are hard or impossible for me to do. I want this dream badly. I know I'll be able to be a really good minister. But I've already failed two classes even though I'm trying.

I have to take them. What if I don't pass them? What will I do if I can't graduate? I pray for help, because I can't do this without help.

LISA'S STORY: HEALING THE WOUNDS WITHIN

Although you like what you do for a living, you feel a nagging lack of confidence and low self-esteem that's been with you since you were a kid. That's how Lisa feels all the time.

In the fourth grade there was a girl named Karla. She was so sweet. She could be quiet and she could sit still, and all her teachers loved her. She never even had to try to get people to like her.

I dreamed of being like Karla. But I never even made it into the classroom. I was always acting up, getting into a fight with someone, not paying attention, and doing things that would keep me from getting my work done. At home I was the one everyone pointed at and said, "You're weird."

It's still that way. I'm still learning how to shut out things that distract me. It's hard for me to stay with one thing. When I got my own talk show, it was great to be on the air because there was a lot to hold my attention. But preparing for the show was something else. I'd get distracted at home going through all the latest local and national newspapers because I couldn't concentrate on one story at a time.

I feel like I'll never be at the same level everybody else is on. I'm always behind. My world is painful. It used to be so painful that I got into a lot of stuff that I shouldn't have to tone down the pain. I'm better now, but emotionally I still have to work with the pain. I wonder if I'll ever feel okay.

TITUS'S STORY: HOPE FOR A NEW LIFE

Have you made so many mistakes in life that you don't see how you'll ever be able to succeed? And now, once again, even though you're trying, you're about to be busted for not being able to control your behavior? That's what happened to Titus.

All I said to my GED teacher was, "Hey man! I'm not trying to cause you trouble." It was then that she threatened to send me to the "hole."

I may be wearing prison khakis, but I'm not all bad. Just because I rock my chair back and forth and get up and down all the time doesn't mean I'm being disrespectful. I just can't sit still. Besides, rocking helps me think.

All I've ever done was try to help others. I dropped out of school when I was 15 when our mom walked out on us. I had to work so my little sister could stay in school and we could eat. It didn't take long to figure out that I couldn't make enough money for a room, food, clothes, and all the stuff you need to survive. So I started to sell drugs. That way we could make it. And my sister stayed in school.

Now I've got a little boy of my own who I only get to see on visitation days. I want something better for him. I'll sure never leave him. I want my GED so I can teach him when I get out of here. I'll make sure my family has what it needs. Sometimes, though, I get just as scared as I did when my mom left. What if I fail?

JASON'S STORY: THE MIDDLE PATH

Are you emotionally lost, like having no idea who you are or what you like or where you're going even though you've tried your whole life to be a good person? That's how Jason feels.

When I was a kid I remember trying real hard to do things right, but somehow I never succeeded. I never achieved the results my family expected from me. I learned to be quiet. I sort of faded into the background—that way I didn't feel so guilty.

My parents helped me a lot. My dad got me into the right schools even though I didn't have the grades. Later, he introduced me to friends so I could get the right jobs. My mom saw that I attended the right social events to match their expectations for me. But I never fit into any of this.

I'm not doing any better now that I'm married and have kids. I don't seem to please my wife, who is much more in charge of what's happening for us than I am. Basically, I am depressed all the time and see no way out. I have to keep pretending. I can't let my family down. But life sure isn't much fun. I guess it never will be.

1

WHAT IS ADD? YOUR CHOICE

Each of us has the opportunity to decide how we want to define ADD. If this sounds odd, read on. How do you want to think about yourself . . . your brain construction? What do you want to do about how you are made? You have a choice. You can see yourself as *disordered*: "There's something wrong with me." Or you can see yourself as a representative of diversity: "I am the way I was made, and that's just fine."

There is not a right or wrong choice. But how you believe about yourself and what you choose to do about it will depend upon the choices you make. Once you become aware that you have a choice, you become in control of what you do and how you feel about yourself. Because you're in control, your self-esteem will rise. What a nice reward for taking charge of your belief-making. It's up to you. No authority or professional can define such things for you. You get to be the boss.

HISTORY OF ADD DEFINITIONS

Despite my urging you to take charge of what you choose to believe, you will bump into lots of pressure from the outside world to believe in one way. One standard operating belief has been designed by professionals in psychiatry, psychology, and mental health. The official diagnosis has changed over time. I am going to give you a brief historical timeline that I've taken from the Diagnostic and Statistical Manual (DSM) of the American Psychiatric Association from 1980 to the present.

- Prior to 1980, ADD in adults was considered to be a childhood condition that was outgrown.

- 1980: The belief stated that a few children with diagnosed ADD continue to show signs of the illness in adulthood without periods of remission.

- 1987: *Undifferentiated Attention Deficit Disorder is a category of disturbances in which the predominant feature is the persistence of developmentally inappropriate and marked inattention that is not a symptom of any other disorder.*

- 1992: When I first wrote about ADD in adults, I presented a definition that reflected the way I was trained. It was primarily shaped by the medical model that looked at ADD as a disorder—something was wrong with the person who "*had it*."

- 1997: The definition I quoted in the third edition of this book had changed little: *Attention Deficit Disorder is a debilitating, little-recognized, and widespread condition.*

You'll notice that words such as *illness, debilitating*, and *symptom* are used, reflecting the medical model upon which they are based. Of course, the very name chosen for ADD/ADHD, Attention Deficit *Disorder*, defines it as an *abnormal condition.*

Also, slowly, throughout these years, the definition changed from that of a disorder only afflicting children, to one in which a few people continue to show symptoms of ADD in adulthood, to one believed to continue into adulthood.

By 1997, I'd become uncomfortable with the medical model as a defining framework for ADD. My strong background in healthy child and adult development led me to realize that there was considerable diversity in the way in which people are made: physically, emotionally, and mentally.

In my speaking and then in my writing (*A.D.D. and Creativity*, 1997), I was expressing ADD as a *type* or *style* of brain wiring rather than a disorder or even the reflection of a *deficit.* I was not even comfortable calling it a *difference* because all people are different—people with a linear type of brain construction are equally different from those with an ADD (nonlinear or analog) style of brain construction. But linear people do not need to say they are different. I was beginning to realize that brainstyle is a diversity issue, not an issue of a *disorder* that needs *treatment*. Training can be useful when a person with ADD attributes must function in a linear setting just as training can be useful when a linear person must function in a nonlinear setting.

MY PREFERRED DEFINITION

By late 1997, the definition of ADD I favored was:

> ADD is a neurobiochemical style of brain wiring.

No judgments and no negative connotations were included in this statement of fact. The only change I've made since that time is to drop the mention of "neurobiochemical wiring":

> ADD is simply a style of brain construction.

I continue to see that:

> This particular style of brain construction, called Attention Deficit Disorder, affects the ways in which we think, feel, create, process information, learn best, manage time, organize projects and materials, respond to our environment, communicate, act physically, and relate to others.

People with ADD do not do these things in a wrong way. We just do them in ways that are not linear. This also means we do not do things that are always compatible with the values held by traditional Western culture.

Gaining acceptance for a definition for ADD that reflects natural diversity rather than being pathological has been very hard. Acceptance has been slow in coming, especially in the professional community. There is a lot of work yet to do by both those of us with significant ADD attributes as well as those who have few such attributes. Yet honoring diversity of brainstyles will not only free the wonderful potential held by those labeled ADD, but also will provide the world with the blessings inherent whenever diversity is respected. We will all benefit from the resulting teamwork that utilizes all brainstyles, creating more than twice the outcome than one preferred style can hope to achieve by itself.

It makes me wonder how in the world the whole ADD business became so "medicalized" and "pathologized." A study of Western history, belief systems, and power structures is necessary to gain a full answer. This is yet to be done.

My observation is that people who like to study and label the way people are made tend to have a brain construction that favors a linear, step-by-step approach. Otherwise they would have little interest in organizing and labeling bits of information. I don't wish to criticize all people with other brainstyles than mine. But I do need to point out that those who tend to do the kind of research that comes up with labels for "pathological" conditions, those who created the label ADD/ADHD and call it a disorder, don't understand about natural human differences. The conclusion they have arrived at is "People different from us are abnormal."

I can only laugh at the thought of one of us with a nonlinear (ADD) brainstyle trying to create a diagnostic and statistical manual. Such an imaginary scenario would make good stand-up comedy material. It's as unlikely as a linear person willingly doing improvisation at a moment's notice with accompanying comedic antics.

CHOOSING FOR OURSELVES

You are faced with how to *believe* about the way you're made.

The choices range from seeing yourself as someone who is in need of fixing to seeing yourself as someone with favorable and valuable assets that are useful and needed in society, so much so that you wouldn't want to change a thing about yourself. It is your choice how to believe. The choice of how to proceed from here is also yours. By applying the three-pronged approach to living with ADD, you can come to feel good about the True You, the way you were innately made, to heal aspects of yourself that have been wounded because of being ADD, and to develop skills that will help you make accommodations to the world in which you live that don't require you to forsake the True You.

Even if you don't want to change the way you are, you may wish to gain assistance to do what doesn't fit you. Know that it doesn't matter whether you are primarily a nonlinear person or a linear one, such assistance is needed to reach outside of your natural scope of abilities.

You must be firm enough and powerful enough to believe in yourself as you are naturally constructed, if your brainstyle is not the socially acceptable style. Blacks in our culture have faced this same challenge, as have women and other "minorities" or segments of our population that are not in favor.

The older definitions of yourself as *disordered* carry the notion that you need to be "fixed." They also give hope that, with "fixing," you will be able to "pass" in the linear culture. It's important to reach a time when you no longer need to hide how you are made—but you can still gain help to ameliorate the effects of ADD wounding and accommodate the status quo without confessing that you are inadequate.

The choice is yours. I've come to the point that I do not wish to say what is right for you in this regard. That would be like telling you what to believe. But feel supported in knowing all people are valuable. All brainstyles are valuable. All decisions are valuable. Know, too, that you are in charge of your beliefs, and inherent in your choices is your power to find peace and self-acceptance.

ALTERNATIVE CHOICES

Finding peace and self-acceptance is easier said than done. But it's possible. First, you must decide where you want the power and control over your life to lie. There is truly no one right answer.

Ask yourself if you're more comfortable fitting into a structure or belief system that is already in place. That's what LaShawna did.

LaShawna's beliefs from her past must be taken into account as she gently and slowly changes some of them so she can escape the negative, self-depreciating perception of herself. To do this, she needs structure and step-by-step support. A medication regimen can help provide what she needs at this time.

If LaShawna's story is familiar to you, you can ask yourself the following questions: Do you like the idea of being a part of a group or structure, including a work team or company? Do you like being identified with a group that has specific beliefs that are shared by all the members? Belonging may make you feel proud or secure. When you weigh the requirements of the group/organization or situation in relation to what you want for yourself, do you come out feeling pretty much okay?

You may not share all the beliefs held by a group, but remain a member, anyway. I don't seem to be able to do that if the group has a shared belief I don't share. Neither of our choices is right or wrong. We simply have different needs and desires.

If you chafe at the needs or demands of the group, you may want to rethink what you're getting in return. Consider whether you still want to be a part of that situation. I have increasingly chosen to concentrate on my strengths and team up with others to cover my weaknesses, while pretty much staying out of structured settings. For example, I no longer do work assignments developed by others. Instead, I focus on creating programs I want to create and writing what I want to write. Then I find someone or some organization that wants to use what I have. Even with the Texas Forest Service, a structured state agency, I don't take assignments but rather come up with ideas

LaShawna's Story: Embracing An ADD Diagnosis

LaShawna has a job that she clings to, even though she doesn't get promoted. Worse yet, she told her counselor, "My employer made me do work I wasn't hired to do. I was hired to file and make copies. Then he told me I had to work the reception desk. Coworkers complained I screwed up the computer all the time."

Whining, she continued, "How could I be expected to keep track of all the details? But, I had to keep the job."

Angrily, she added, "I don't have the luxury to look for another job."

"Can you believe what happened next? I went for career guidance, and the counselor said I am wimpy, whiny, and have a low energy level. Besides that, he said people with my degree are a dime a dozen."

"Well, that sure made me mad." LaShawna then began telling how she was taking a graduate class at the university and had found a part-time job tutoring in the disabilities center. But that didn't turn out very well, either. Her boss told LaShawna she caused more trouble than any other tutor. It seems one of her students worked at a low level and LaShawna complained about it and refused to work with the student any longer. In fact, she decided she would never again work with anyone who has a disability.

She further complained that the student shouldn't have been admitted in the first place because she "wasn't fit to do college work." Irritably, she moaned, "Even a high school dropout realizes disabled students are not to get a free ride on the gravy train." Needless to say, her anger, petulance, and scolding tone didn't endear her to her boss. She wasn't welcomed back the next semester.

It was then that someone she knew casually mentioned she'd like to go to a lecture on ADD. LaShawna decided to go, too, though she didn't expect to get much out of it. To her surprise, she quickly identified with the characteristics of ADD without Hyperactivity. At age fifty, she finally found an explanation for some of the problems she had encountered all her life: short-term memory deficit, being scatterbrained, experiencing trouble doing more than one thing at a time, and having lots of sensitivity. She thought, "No wonder I've been so depressed all the time and couldn't organize and manage details."

She began to believe she could change the way she is made. Then maybe she'd be able to get a job and keep it—one that even has benefits. She immediately tried medication and went to the school's memory center to get help for her problem with details. She also started seeing a counselor who works especially with mature people who only recently discovered they have ADD—people whose lifestyles had become entrenched in beliefs about their lack of worth and inadequacy.

The counselor quickly noticed LaShawna's high level of anger and negative approach to new ideas when he tried to guide her toward jobs and graduate work that better fit her unique skills and abilities. LaShawna had spent too many years believing poorly about herself to entertain another way of doing things.

Progress was slow, but a little light occasionally shone in LaShawna's eyes as she spoke of liking to write and do research. Then she qualified her statement with, "But I'm sure I can't get a job writing." After a moment, she thinks of a second reason she can't do what she wants to do: "You have to have a lot of schooling, more than I have, to do research."

Although it will take a while for LaShawna to broaden her horizons, she is showing signs that she is breaking through her captivity and is being redirected toward something different than she's known. She's insistent the medication for her ADD brainstyle will help her. Perhaps it will, though it won't help the years of learned helplessness and accumulation of a negative self-image.

LaShawna has not seen that more of her problems are due to her negative approach to people than to ADD. But because having a label to explain her problems gives her an opportunity to hope for change, especially with medication usage, LaShawna may have opened a door that will allow her to actually see her True Self.

There's no doubt that LaShawna does better in structured situations at this time in her life. With the buildup of anger and negative thinking, low self-confidence, little practical experience in the work world, and no clear picture of what's unique about herself, LaShawna needs time to fill in the deficits in herself. She could even learn about living in the world if she is willing to work at it.

Finding her fit is not much of an option for her—at least not until she believes enough in herself to stand up for her feelings. She must find new ways to make herself feel valuable, even in situations that don't fit her brainstyle. So LaShawna will need all the help she can get at this time. That means structure and treatment for her ADD-style brain.

The relief she feels at embracing an ADD diagnosis and treatment are giving her new hope. And hope makes her feel better than she has ever felt before in her life. Maybe she will eventually be able to dream.

to fill the needs the agency has—ideas that interest me, too. But this choice is not for everyone.

Sometimes we outgrow a traditional setting. It may have served us well initially or for a long time, but then we become ready to spread our wings and try out new territory.

Sam has both chosen freedom to pursue the interests of his True Self and reached for the structure through school that would balance his desire for self-employment.

Sam's Story: Taking a Little of This and That

Sam's success is in large part the outgrowth of his mother's comment, "I don't worry about him anymore."

"You can succeed and be happy whether your brainstyle fits the mainstream or not," says his mom now that she's changed her perception of her son from one that focused on his problems to one that focuses on his strengths and gifts.

Sam's life was not always so happy. It didn't promise success. In fact, misery would be a more apt description from age seven to age sixteen. Unable to read in second grade, he was called "stupid" by his classmates. In third grade, he was diagnosed with Attention Deficit Disorder with Hyperactivity, and in fifth grade Sam's parents found themselves totally confused and terribly fearful for Sam.

What were they to do? What happened to the bright, delightful child of many colors who was their son?

His reading continued to be an insurmountable problem, but at the end of fifth grade, his school system had created a dyslexia program. He began to get extra help with his attentional problems. But school continued to cause great difficulties. He appeared to do anything to avoid doing homework. His mother and father worried about what would happen to Sam in high school and whether he'd ever be able to make a living as an adult.

Sam's problems labeled, his parents felt better, but still they worried. Then one day, his mother met a woman who'd worked with people with ADD for many years. Hearing that Sam had been diagnosed with ADD, the woman looked intently at Sam's mother. To the mother's surprise, instead of asking what his problem was, she asked, "What does your son love to do?"

The mother, momentarily taken aback, finally said softly, "He loves to fish and to play guitar." When the ADD counselor met Sam, he told her in depth about his last fishing trip. She was wide-eyed with all he knew, not only about the process of fishing, but also about the fish themselves. At sixteen, he could also manage to pilot a deep-sea fishing boat with clients who wanted to do gulf fishing on their vacations. He brought out his 12-string guitar, and she saw the light in his eye and heard the music his skillful fingers produced.

She clearly remembers turning to the parents and saying, "Don't you ever worry about this young man again. He will be fine. He is wonderful. Sure, school will be messy, but he'll get through it and find his way."

Sam's mother believed her. She felt relief. Because of that one comment, she started to get her husband, family, and friends to accept her son for the kind of unique individual he is and provide the kind of support that would open options for his life. She even came to believe that "If passing school is not a part of that, we could still survive."

As of this writing, Sam has been on his own for over five years. During his junior year in high school, Sam began to have hope, too. As a result of an Internet networking class, he was given the opportunity to immediately apply what he was learning as he learned it. He made the highest grade in the class. Sam went to work at an Internet company full-time when he graduated and stayed there for four years, performing increasingly complicated tasks and taking on more responsibility. At that point, Sam felt he'd learned all there was to learn, "at that company," so he decided to go into business for himself. And he entered college to take one class. He felt ready to try formal education again.

Though his mother's worries resurfaced for a short period, they quickly disappeared as Sam sought the legitimate help he needed to conquer a difficult class. He is happy with being in school and making a good grade in the class. He now believes he can learn in school.

Most important of all, Sam sees himself realistically, which allows for him to enjoy and use his gifts while choosing how to accommodate his weaknesses. He's chosen to do the kinds of work he likes and does well. He talks to teachers about getting the kind of accommodations he needs. He asks his parents or friends for help with written material as needed. He's chosen not to take medication for his ADD. Instead, he reads while walking around or takes breaks to play his guitar when he feels restless.

Sam has taken his mother's advice to focus on what he does well instead of what he doesn't do well. His glass is half full.

Sam's self-awareness, perseverance, and attitude about himself guarantee not only a future for him, but also one in which he can model the value of respecting and honoring diversity, no matter what it looks like.

If Sam's story sounds familiar to you, you may wish to ask yourself some questions. "Do I want to march to the beat of my own drum while at the same time feeling the support of something regular and consistent in my life? Am I in a place in my life where I am sure-footed enough to allow myself to try new things? Do I know how to get help when I need it? Do I know when I need it?"

Sometimes those of us who like to fly free and have little external control over us find a time when we do seek out structure. When our lives come under stress, we are more likely to want to have something stable upon which to lean. If we are brand new at doing something or tired or feeling "old," if we've suffered a loss or have had a number of changes in our lives,

Alisha's Story: On-Again, Off-Again ADD

As the daughter of a riverboat captain and the boat's social director, Alisha spent the first eight years of her life with the deck hands and crew as her extended family, teachers, and friends. Beached and sent to Catholic school, she felt as if she'd been placed in a cage. Needless to say, Alisha didn't like school very much. The first ADD red flags went up in fourth grade, when she "blew the ceiling off the aptitude tests" but did poorly on routine tests and homework assignments—which she rarely turned in. Throughout the remaining years of school and college she did okay, but didn't "live up to her potential."

Once out of the educational system, she blossomed. Her work life was exemplary. She taught high school and coached for fifteen years and earned a master's degree in educational administration. She served as an assistant principal to a principal who thought well of her. But she hated being a disciplinarian, and the teachers were "always on her tail" because of late paperwork.

Tired out from doing a job she really didn't want to do, she returned to school to receive training in her beloved field, counseling and guidance. With a degree in hand, she happily returned to the workplace and thrived, often working with kids in alternative schools and others who were hard to reach. And was she ever effective!

With retirement, she spent time developing her singing and storytelling. She'd played guitar since she was in seventh grade and enjoyed entertaining as an adult.

Personal events took a downward turn, however, and Alisha made a startling discovery. With no history of regular attendance at church, she went with a friend to hear a woman minister preach in another town. She heard how there was a shortage of ministers, especially women in the ministry. The lightbulb went off, and six months later she had her interview for acceptance in seminary based largely upon her excellent work history. She excitedly began to study.

Returning to school turned out to be hell. Now ready to begin her third year, she reports several failures in difficult subjects that are very linear in nature. She's also having trouble getting her assignments done in a timely manner, which creates more failure. Last summer, she went into the field and once again thrived, performing her assignment with excellence. Next, she was able to take her internship early (before the end of her third year), working in a small town church where she is happy, successful, and well liked. She has both a vision for the year and her dream for when she gets out of seminary.

But before Alisha can implement her dream, she will need to finish the third year of school and pass a class she's failed twice. She does have plans for succeeding. Guided by her work with a mental health clinician, Alisha has begun to feel better about herself. She sought help with her depression and with ADD. This gave her a new perspective on her ability to learn, and her depression lifted.

At the end of her second year, she has found other students who also need help with ADD and other learning differences. By talking with them, she has begun to feel her own power building. In conversations with her academic dean, she has found out that he wants to help her with her learning difficulties but doesn't know what to do.

Her job, with the help of other interested students and outside professionals, is to prepare to educate the dean and faculty. She plans to request accommodation for an intervention involving her Greek translation class. Though there is a computerized program available to translate Greek texts to English, Alisha's degree program requires her to be able to translate the material directly. She has failed the class twice and does not know how she can possibly pass. She and another ADD student need to be allowed to translate the texts using whatever method works for them. Then they can use the content appropriately in their ministry.

Alisha plans to suggest a specialist in ADD visit with the dean to talk about what is reasonable accommodation for someone with her brainstyle. Then the dean can pass the information on to the professor so the goal of translation can be achieved and Alisha and her classmate can get on with the business of ministering.

I hope Alisha's dreams work out for her. She is dedicated, and she is strong in the people skills required of ministers. She conceptualizes a nontraditional ministry using her guitar playing and singing at retreats that she would like to hold in the great Texas out of doors. I can clearly visualize the creative ministry she describes—a vision that even includes her plying her craft much as circuit riders once did. And I know, despite her on-again, off-again ADD problem—a problem that only shows up in traditional educational settings and rarely when she's actually working—Alisha is going to make good as a minister lady.

aligning ourselves with a definite order can feel mighty good. We may choose to introduce structure into a small part of our lives, finding this is enough to ground us so we can regain our balance.

As the consequence of where we are in our need or desire for structure, whether it's permanent or transitory, we must become aware of what will make us feel comfortable and help us be more productive and responsible. To that end, the way we look at our particular style of brain construction will determine how we want to deal with it.

At present, the majority approach is to consider ADD as a *disorder* requiring remediation. What I want to do in this book is open up the option of finding and going with your True Self, healing your Wounded Self, and teaching your Accommodating Self as a response to your ADD style. By choosing to consider ADD as a natural, perfectly normal style of brain construction, by healing your wounds, and by focusing on finding schooling, a lifestyle, and jobs that fit, you will not only cease being *disabled*, but will also use to advantage the skills and talents with which you were born.

A MIDDLE PATH

You do not need to take an all-or-nothing approach to the way in which you look at and respond to ADD. Find the right balance for you. You may realize that there is nothing wrong with the way you are, but let's say you have to spend time in a school setting that was not designed with your brainstyle in mind. You will likely find you are at a distinct disadvantage. You might not even be able to get through school to get the credential or license you need in order to do a job that is beautifully suited to you.

Do you function fine with people, understand their needs, communicate well, and conjure loyalty? Do you have a dream that requires formal school? If so, are you frightened that you may not be able to make the grades you need to get your credential or degree? Do you know what to do but just don't test well in order to prove that you know the material?

If you answer "yes" to these questions, you may need to look into formal accommodation through the Americans with Disabilities Act (see appendix D). Every school has student services that can provide you with reasonable accommodation by law. If you take advantage of these, keep in mind that you could learn what you need to learn in ways that fit you, but there just doesn't happen to be an apprenticeship or kinesthetic program available to teach you in the way that you naturally learn.

2

IDENTIFICATION VERSUS DIAGNOSIS OF ADD

It does not take a rocket scientist to identify ADD characteristics in yourself or in another. Never in forty years of counseling, child development, and human behavior work have I seen as high a level of accurate self-recognition as I have with Attention Deficit Disorder. If you identify with what you read from a list of attributes of ADD, you can be sure you are a person with an ADD style of brain construction. (See appendix A for the "New ADD Assessment Checklist.")

Because there are no exact criteria for ADD, it can't be said that you "have *it*" or you "don't have *it*." Instead, you will have more or fewer ADD attributes. It's not a black-and-white issue any more than skin color is. Some folks have lots and lots of ADD attributes, while others have almost none. And a whole bunch of people have some ADD attributes and some linear attributes and fall in the middle of a brainstyle. I call these folks "bridge people." They are useful at helping people with opposite brainstyles to communicate and work together.

John Rubel, who wrote the foreword for this book, and I are a case in point. We took the same ADD assessment in a workshop. He scored two points and I scored 58. The more points, the more ADD attributes you have. We laughed, already knowing that we were nearly polar opposites. And when we talk, as we often do, we have to carefully explain our meanings to each other so that we end up on the same page. Of course, the more we've gotten to know one another, the more each automatically factors meaning into the other's responses because we understand the backdrop upon which our communications are silhouetted.

It is possible, though unnecessary, to spend hundreds and even thousands of dollars to arrive at an ADD diagnosis. Interestingly, the word *diagnosis* is associated with ADD when the expensive medical model is used to identify an ADD style of brain construction. Lengthy interviews, brain scans, and psychological tests will tell you about how you're constructed, but they aren't necessary to identify an ADD brainstyle.

The term *dual diagnosis* is frequently introduced when lengthy diagnostic workups are involved. Inherent in this term is the assumption that ADD is pathological, creating the dual aspect of diagnosis.

Neither is ADD a "diagnosis of exclusion." You don't have to screen out every other form of physical, cognitive, and emotional state to end up with a definitive diagnosis of ADD. You can have an innate ADD brainstyle with all sorts of physical, cognitive, and emotional strengths and impairments. Similarly, you can have all sorts of physical, cognitive, and emotional strengths and impairments with a linear brainstyle.

ADD will have been present since birth, will remain through puberty, and will continue intact until you die. You don't acquire it somewhere along the way.

There are checklists galore, but they each have several features in common. The biggest problem with the majority of the checklists is that they are value laden and judgmental. In the behaviors and attributes they list, they frequently reflect the secondary wounding attributes of ADD created by environments that don't fit. I discovered this phenomenon when I led workshops on "Brainstyle Diversity in Action." These were conducted among settings including women's groups, prison professionals, and students.

Each participant in the workshop filled out a standard paper-and-pencil ADD checklist. Next, each participant was placed in one of three groups: ADD people, bridge people, and linear people. Each group worked as a team on tasks that were analog (nonlinear), linear, and a combination of both. I did not anticipate the results that I got.

When the ADD group was given a linear task, such as ordering the members of their group by foot size, they never really achieved the result. They spent their time telling stories that related to their feet and shoes. They never got around to ordering themselves by foot size. The linear folks took about two minutes to quietly rank themselves in a sequential line from largest foot size to smallest foot size. The bridge people only took a little longer than the linear people, but they laughed more.

The ADD group lived up to their reputation by failing to achieve the goal and becoming raucous, disorderly, restless, and inattentive. There were even a few wet eyes as they shared tales of sensitive memories taken from early life around the issue of foot size.

However, when the groups were assigned a nonlinear (analog) task such as designing a program that would communicate to the public about the many faces of ADD, the linear group became raucous, disorderly, restless, and inattentive. They spoke out impulsively. They also became emotional, though their emotions were more those of irritation and even anger than withdrawal and tears. They discounted the assignment ("What a waste of time") rather than expressing feelings of inadequacy ("I can't do this"). They also didn't complete the task.

The bridge people had some ideas and were adequate to the task, but not visionary. They tried to think of ways to implement what they understood to be the goal. They reported feeling torn between wanting to think "outside of the box" and "getting something on paper" in the time allotted.

Interesting to me was the way in which the ADD people tackled the nonlinear task. They demonstrated considerable attention, saw the big picture, and even began to break the implementation down into manageable bits. They were active, often talking with their hands and even walking around acting out how a public awareness activity could be accomplished. All of their activity had meaning. They role-played their plans and stuck with the task until their program was fleshed out and ready to be implemented.

When the ADD folks had carried the activity as far as they wanted, they turned to the bridge group and asked them to help with the actual details of implementation. What I observed was the building of a team. They veered away from asking for help from the linear people. Perhaps this had to do with previous experiences trying to work with people with that brainstyle, or perhaps they were put off by the critical, angry expressions they observed in the workshop. I did not ask them.

With this in mind, I began to see the lists of ADD symptoms in a different light. I realized that most of the so-called symptoms of ADD are behavioral symptoms that appear when people with an ADD brainstyle are assigned linear tasks. They do not apply when their assignment or attention is directed to works and tasks that fit their particular brainstyle.

CRITIQUE OF TRADITIONAL ADD SYMPTOM LISTS

Let's consider several behaviors that are generally attributed to people with ADD:

Difficulty with attention/focusing. No distinction is made with regard to the kind of situation in which the attention and focusing are directed. When Sam plays his 12-string guitar, he pays a lot of attention. When Lisa is interviewing a guest on her talk show, she focuses intently on the theme of the interview and has no problem attending even to the multitasking details of running the talk show segment.

People with an ADD brainstyle have often been accused of concentrating on tasks they *like* to do, as if that verifies that they are deficient or abnormal. This is actually no different than what happens with linear people who are doing tasks that do or don't fit them. We all *like* to do what fits us and *don't like* to do what doesn't.

Overfocusing. Again, I would ask about the setting in which the overfocusing occurs. Generally, overfocusing means a person is immersed in a task so deeply that he or she does not respond to requests to do something else. This assumes that there is a "right" amount of time to focus on or accomplish a task. Because people with ADD tend to become a part of what they are doing in a personal way, they tend to want to carry the task to completion. It's beyond me how this way of focusing is abnormal. It's nothing more than a style of focusing attention.

In contrast, sometimes the amount of time allotted for a task is more than the time it takes the ADD person to do the task. Both disconnecting from a task prematurely and pretending to stay involved past the time that is beneficial for the completion of the task are frustrating and difficult for ADD folks.

Some of us prefer to work in smaller segments. We work until our minds have exhausted themselves or we've used up the thought material that we have at that time. Then we break, do something else, and return when the coffers of our mind have new material to contribute to the completion of the task.

There is nothing *wrong* with or *pathological* about this way of working. It's just different from the way linear folks may approach a task. Part of the difference comes from the kinesthetic (hands-on) manner ADD people use for task completion. We *live* a task. So, if we're teaching, we become immersed in teaching, bringing the subject alive. The more linear approach tends to teach *about* a subject, not really living it but talking or demonstrating *about* it. This difference is often misread by people who don't understand the diversity of thinking styles.

Difficulty with activity level (hyperactivity, hypoactivity, or restlessness). There is no question that most of us with ADD move a lot, think a lot, and/or talk a lot. But why is movement considered unacceptable and less conducive to learning than stillness? It is only a problem if we are required to learn or work in a sedate manner. Who said it is normal or necessary to sit down in a cramped school desk in order to learn to read?

What happened to the apprenticeship model of learning? It fits nonlinear processors perfectly. I do not see how activity level can be judged to be too much or too little.

When examining hypoactivity, I look at what preceded the decline in activity. I've found that upon questioning, the individual who is "just sitting there" may be thinking. Some of us think through a problem, situation, or request completely before making a move, and then the resultant activity comes out in a whole unit. This is quite different from the gluing together of one detail or step to the next and then to the next, ad infinitum, in order to build a thought or product such as an essay. Big-picture people just don't do things that way.

Difficulty with hypersensitivity (mood variability and reactivity). How much sensitivity is too much? Have we come to a time in history where being emotionally touched by the events, problems, and people around us is considered wrong or pathological? I wonder how much is too much or too little. Perhaps undersensitivity is as big a problem as, or an even bigger problem than, oversensitivity.

Yes, people with an ADD style of brain construction tend to be sensitive to what is going on around them. It's like having acute sensors that pick up the energy of people's emotions, social trends, and just about anything and everything that is in the environment. But what they are feeling also tends to be very real, that is, there is something present or happening. Getting your feelings hurt by hurtful words and actions seems like a pretty healthy response to me. I've often observed the person who is saying, "You're too sensitive," is actually very insensitive. Why label one side of the behavioral exchange and not the other? Or better yet, why label either?

Like the canary that dies from gas poisoning before the humans around realize there is a danger, ADD people will often sense external cues long before the person with few ADD characteristics has an awareness of what is going on. There's also the analogy drawn from gardenias that turn brown when their petals are touched. Is the gardenia oversensitive, disordered, or judged to be wrong? No. That just happens to be how gardenias and canaries are made. It's neither right nor wrong. And neither are people with an ADD style of brain construction disordered because they are sensitive.

Mood variability is similar to sensitivity. Generally, any change in your emotions is due to a change in your relationship to the environment around you. Sensitivity to external energy leads to changing moods. If you are in a room with hostility or anger, it's likely that you'll feel the results and become either hostile and angry or fearful and withdrawn, both of which are protections against what's going on around you. To be told you're too sensitive makes no sense.

Another source of mood variability comes from the fact that living in a culture that generally does not allow for brainstyle diversity is a painful thing for the "out" group. Fraught with experiences of failure, this group may wildly celebrate any success, even minor ones. From the depression of failure to the joy of success! Add to that the ability to feel deeply, and you get broad emotions over a wide range.

People who are constructed differently just don't understand. All these feelings may even frighten them. The result is they label the difference as a problem, not realizing that it is only a problem for them, not an inherent problem. Labeling is unnecessary. Acceptance of diversity is much more constructive.

Talking about reactiveness, a lot is said about the importance of not getting emotionally involved with your work. There is a myth out there that it is possible to be "objective" about one's work. Unfortunately, no matter how anyone tries, our biases, beliefs, perceptions, and emotions do play a role in anything and everything we observe or do.

Reactions can be subtle, so it is easy not to see them. Or they can be visible. They tend to be visible with ADD people. Either way, reactiveness to all outside stimuli must be factored into every experience.

Difficulty with organization of time, details, and paperwork or the breaking of projects into small segments. When linear organization is expected of ADD people, the result isn't pretty. But when analog organization techniques are used, it turns out they work. For example, keeping projects in stacks on the floor works well for people with ADD. This may not sit well with non-ADD people, just as a messy desk is judged negatively. Often ADD people are told, "You can't find anything that way." But that is not true.

Details do create a problem, especially when a person is expected to start a job by putting the details together in a line. Big-picture people don't work that way. Rather than using details as building blocks, they create or envision a general picture of the job and then find the details as needed or desired. This is only a difference in approach.

The whole issue of breaking projects into small bits smacks of a belief that this is the way to accomplish a task. But if you're a big-picture person, that isn't a useful way to proceed. It also won't happen. Spend time letting the big picture fill out and then ask, "What is the first part of this big picture I want to work with?" The ADD person will sense or feel an answer. And the process will have begun.

Temper. Most temper "problems" of ADD folk are the result of frustration from being expected to act in ways that don't fit, or the result of having your sensitive boundaries crossed. By the time a child is a preschooler, much damage will have been done.

When the birth process takes place in a setting that lacks warmth and personal connection, ADD babies feel the impersonality and coldness. When a baby experiences the roughness of a low thread count in crib sheets, agitation and discomfort set in. When loud noises hurt you and when those around you don't understand why, you blow up from being shamed. It's no wonder that there's a gigantic accumulation of hurt and abuse that occurs, though often unintended, early in life. A child who fights back but is rarely heard escalates his or her expression of discomfort in an attempt to stop the hurting.

Often, though, secondary abuse sets in as a child is scolded or punished because of a reaction to the original abuse. In contrast, when a child is heard, and taught other ways to get his or her needs met, such as verbally, then much of the temper abates. Few people recognize that something needs to be done with sensitive people, and even fewer know what to do if they recognize the need.

When we look closely at the items used to define ADD, it becomes apparent that they are judgmental and value laden. Lack of understanding and self-serving judgment, though not intended, run rampant through the criteria for Attention Deficit Disorder. I would like to substitute the following, more positive, list of ADD characteristics that *do* distinguish people with this particular brainstyle from people who have few ADD characteristics.

NEW LIST OF ATTRIBUTES OF ATTENTION DEFICIT DISORDER

Following are characteristics that describe the makeup of a person with Attention Deficit Disorder. Remember, ADD isn't something you have or don't have. You have more or fewer

ADD characteristics. The more ADD characteristics you have, the more you are likely to:

See the big picture. Many of us see the big picture before we see or make use of any of the details that make it up. Usually creative by nature, big-picture people often see a complete vision of what we want to achieve before we start moving toward our goals. We don't travel toward any goal unless we are provided with the big picture to begin with.

Think in terms of how things function. If we are to know how to proceed toward a goal, we must know its purpose and function. How is this goal to be used? Rather than seeing the details that make up the task, we see the function the details play and the relationships between them. Then we can know the steps to take to achieve the goal.

Pay attention to the patterns and relationships within the big picture. Our focus tends to be on the relationship between details rather than on the details themselves. We see the interconnections and patterns that are formed between things rather than the elements that make them up.

Express high levels of activity: physical, mental, emotional, and verbal. Naturally invested with lots of energy, we learn, create, and produce best when we are active. Our innate skills seek environments for expression that allow us to be physically active and verbally expressive. Our minds are curious and exploring and often work at lightning speed. After all, we see the big picture first, so we don't need to slowly progress from one detail to another in order to reach a completed picture.

We're also aided by our rapid awareness of patterns that often give us early clues about the journey we are taking. The icing on the cake is the presence of big, broad, expressive emotions that communicate, to us and others, with clarity.

Learn by doing (kinesthetic learning). We naturally learn *through* the process of doing something rather than by reading or listening *about* whatever we are learning. We write a book to learn to write. We don't learn to write a book by studying about writing a book, doing exercises or worksheets, or taking exams detailing the grammar needed in the book. We are completely able to learn any subject or body of professional material, no matter how complex, by utilizing kinesthetic learning methods. That's why the apprenticeship model works well for us.

Have an inner locus of perception and control. Our worldview comes from within ourselves. Our ability to organize, work with time and timing, maintain control over our behavior, and do whatever we need to do is idiosyncratically guided from within ourselves rather than from outside.

We know and sense and can learn to live in a responsible way that yields the same results achieved by our more linear counterparts if we follow what *feels right* to us. We know what to do by listening to our inner drumbeat, not by using a template produced outside of ourselves into which we are expected to fit.

Be sensate by nature, having a high level of sensitivity. Our sensitivity is felt through our senses—sight, sound, taste, smell, and touch—as well as intuition. We are extremely empathetic, our sensors calibrated finely. Liken us to the dog that hears sounds not perceived by the human ear. We sense at a level that not all people can.

We are empathetic and responsive to our environments. We can be wounded when others do not see or sense the source of the wounding, yet we experience it nonetheless. We often can do linear tasks such as editing by using our sensate faculties. Many of us are psychic, though we may not be comfortable with this skill or may not purposely use it.

Have a strong sensing capability. We tend to think first through our ability to sense what is going on rather than by thinking *about* something. We simply *know*, having an inner sensory vision, experience, or intuition. We often feel the sensing physically in our bodies. Once we've perceived an event on a sensory level, we can decide what to do in response. We even store information using this mechanism rather than by categorizing according to the verbal labels in more general use.

Resonate to the rhythmic timing of nature. Rather than responding to an arbitrary scheme to keep track of time, we tend to use natural rhythms and our own internal timing to get things done. We can apply this skill to a project or to getting the rest our bodies need. We may work at night and sleep in the daytime. We may naturally eat at times that vary from a three-meal-a-day schedule.

We rarely break projects down into equal time segments in order to get them done by a certain time; rather, we work when we *feel* creative and don't work when we feel unwilling or hesitant. When our innate timing is allowed to blossom and we are trained to recognize it, we always get things done *on time.* Ironically, even when a stated deadline is passed, it usually works out that the actual time in which we completed a task was better for everyone because of some circumstance we didn't know about. For example, the person we were going to meet was delayed and didn't arrive on time, or a better quality of paper arrived after the initial deadline—paper that improved the print job.

Sometimes we must complete one whole assignment, such as a first writing of a book, before we can produce a higher-quality book by rewriting it one more time. This happens because by *living* the writing of the first book, we grow and see how to bring the project to a higher level. Without the first draft, we wouldn't arrive at the quality we eventually achieve.

This approach is particularly necessary when doing linear work such as nonfiction writing. In contrast, work, which by nature is nonlinear, often comes out as a whole unit with few changes.

AN ADDITIONAL PERSPECTIVE ON CHARACTERISTICS OF ADD

In the latter half of the 1990s, I developed a one-page description of characteristics of people with ADD that took account of personality styles that are reflected in three ways in people with an ADD brainstyle. I have updated this material to reflect my current thinking. It includes general characteristics of ADD. Next the description notes three forms of personality styles and ADD characteristics present naturally in environments that allow for expression of the ADD-way as well as characteristics that are likely to occur when you are placed in a linear environment. The three forms are as follows:

Form 1: Outwardly Expressed ADD: The Active Entertainer

Form 2: Inwardly Directed ADD: The Restless Dreamer

Form 3: Highly Structured ADD: The Conscientious Controller

You may be a mix of two or more forms. And each form lends itself to not only a lifestyle, but also specific jobs that successfully make use of the positive attributes (see chart 2.1).

Chart 2.1. New List of Characteristics of ADD

General Characteristics:

Sees the big picture	Thinks in terms of how things function
Pays attention to patterns and relationships within the big picture	
Expresses high levels of activity: physical, mental, emotional, and verbal	
Learns by doing	Has inner locus of perception and control
Is responsive	Has strong sensing capability
Resonates to the rhythmic timing of nature	

These core ADD characteristics seem to surface in adults in three distinct ways. People with ADD may fall into one of three categories, but they can exhibit a "blend" of two or all three forms.

Form I: Outwardly Expressed ADD: The Active Entertainer
Feelings and behaviors are actively and openly expressed. Many with this form like employment in sales, entertainment, entrepreneurship, or fast-paced and high-energy fields.

Traits:

Outwardly active	Spontaneous	High-risk taker
Wide mood capability	Quick to change	Reacts to external pressure
Highly demonstrative	Multitasks	Expresses temper outwardly
Prefers to break large tasks into segments, creating many small tasks		

In linear situations:

Easily bored	Short attention span	Dislikes long-term projects
Becomes reactive	Dislikes repetition	Blames others when frustrated
Expresses temper		

Form II: Inwardly Directed ADD: The Restless Dreamer
Feelings and behavior are not actively displayed, but internalized or subtly expressed. May like employment in field involving creativity, sensitivity, the out of doors, and mechanics, or service-oriented work.

Traits:

Very empathetic	Sticks to jobs liked	Slow to change
Very sensitive	Visionary/dreamer	Often highly creative
Good problem solver	Prefers freedom to explore	Restless

(continued)

Chart 2.1. *(continued)*

In linear situations:

Tends to blame self	Distractible when bored	Burns out
Tends toward depression	Vacillates	Tries too hard

Form III: Highly Structured ADD: The Conscientious Controller
Must work within a structure. Tends to feel out of control if structure is changed. Emotions are expressed as judgments. Often anxious and demanding. One with this type of ADD can usually succeed in the military, accounting, or a field utilizing computers and attention to detail and precision.

Traits:

Very organized	Likes structure	Perfectionist
Highly focused	Talkative	Dislikes interruptions
Mentally restless	Systematic problem solver	Takes charge in a crisis
Prefers to work a task from beginning to end without a break		

In linear situations:

Demanding	Rigid	Judgmental
Obsessively worries	Loses temper	Controlling

As you can see, there are both general attributes shared by all three forms and specific personality characteristics that differ between the forms. For example, if you have some Form I characteristics, you will tend to want to multitask. If you have Form III characteristics, you will hate multitasking and prefer to stick with a long-term project to the end, once you've started it. In fact, you're likely to fail to get back to it if you take breaks. If your predominant Form is II, then the way you handle tasks, with or without breaks, will be dependent upon the other forms of ADD brainstyle you have. It is also possible that you are a mix of all three.

As you use this descriptive chart, simply circle the items that seem to fit you. Then you will see the predominant tendency within the framework of your ADD brainstyle—a tendency that you prefer to work within. Give yourself permission to follow that urge. You can trust your feelings, remembering that it doesn't matter how you are constructed, just that you honor the way in which you are made.

YOU GET TO CHOOSE

Given this information about the history and various definitions of ADD and criteria for identifying it, you are faced with various ways to decide how you want to look at Attention Deficit Disorder in general and, specifically, in relation to yourself. Each perspective has merits as well as drawbacks.

It's mighty hard to live true to your innate ADD brainstyle in a society that requires linear skills to learn and prove that you can do a job. It's hard to fit into a nine-to-five world when your natural rhythm has you up all night and sleeping in the daytime. It's hard to be sensitive in a harsh environment.

Practically speaking, most of us need to take a three-pronged approach in dealing with our ADD brainstyle. We can believe in ourselves and honor how we are constructed as often as possible while learning what we can do to "fit in." That way, we can achieve a position of power in our society. We must increasingly make our own choices. And that is easier to do when we can both live true to ourselves, doing things in ways that fit our brainstyle, and engage successfully in activities for which we are not particularly suited.

Of great importance: when you choose to veer from using your natural brainstyle, do not believe there is something *wrong* with you, but realize you are making the choice to do what doesn't fit in order to achieve a goal that's important to you. Your Accommodating Self is operating. It's called "Being realistic." But remember, you don't have to see yourself as pathological in order to also be realistic.

3

WHAT ELSE YOU NEED TO KNOW ABOUT ADD

Five frequently asked questions about ADD are:

What causes ADD?

How many people have ADD?

Who has ADD?

Why be concerned about ADD?"

What happens to your emotions when you discover you are ADD?

The first three questions are difficult to answer. However, a brief discussion of each is useful.

WHAT CAUSES ADD?

In this book, I am talking about ADD that appears to have genetic roots. It is easily tracked generation to generation by observing the behavior of family members. The He's-Just-Like-Uncle-George Syndrome.

The roots of Acquired ADD, not covered in this book, are more clearly definable. Environmental factors are one of the culprits of this kind of ADD. Exposure to lead (metal toxicity) is an example. Other conditions that may have ADD components are head injuries, some birth defects and physical syndromes, as well as the aftermath of drug use, such as crack cocaine, a favorite drug for people with ADD who have not made the choices they need to make to get control of their lives.

In earlier editions of this book, this question was derived in relation to the medical model. The question I now prefer is "What causes ADD problems?"

The truth about the initial question, "What causes ADD?" is not known. The research is sketchy, and the studies are generally not well designed. The results also are extremely value laden. For example, results may say, "Something is wrong with the brain . . ." or "Their (people with an ADD style of brain construction) brains seem to be less active, especially in areas controlling concentration and impulsive behavior." But the tasks measured may have been linear tasks. A linear person might have the same difficulty doing a nonlinear task. The research doesn't clearly differentiate the variables being measured.

At one time, family relationships were blamed for the presence of ADD characteristics. This is no longer the case. Other explanations have been forwarded and found lacking, such as poor moral character. Needless to say, extensive, unbiased research is needed if a "cause" or "causes" for ADD are to be unearthed. (See p. 65 for a summary of current research.)

The question, "What causes ADD problems?" elicits a different answer. The primary cause of ADD "problems" is the way in which Western societies have pathologized this normal style of brain construction. The good news is that only the reaction to this style needs to be changed. The bad news is that it's hard to change beliefs and attitudes about anything. Reframing ADD as a diversity issue will mean the general public will have to be given nonjudgmental information and think about what they hear. Once they understand that we're dealing with diversity, those willing to move beyond their prejudices about one style of brain construction being better than another will need to lead a charge to change the conditions that perpetuate the notion of ADD as a disorder.

This means changing institutions, such as education and laws that require ADD to be listed as a "handicapping" condition under the Americans with Disabilities Act, in order to obtain equal opportunity in school and the workplace. It will mean changing the beliefs of the professional community who have made a living researching, diagnosing, and treating ADD.

None of these tasks will be easy, but the reward for individuals and communities will be enormous. The retrieval of an extremely important human resource for the good of all will have been achieved.

HOW MANY PEOPLE HAVE ADD?

With the perspective of ADD forwarded in this book, in which a person doesn't have *it*, but instead has more or fewer ADD attributes, there is no way to determine how many Americans have ADD. With those of us who see ADD as a diversity issue that falls on a continuum of characteristics from more to fewer attributes, the educated guess is that the spread of characteristics falls fairly equally along the continuum.

Other factors also influence the difficulty of determining the number of people involved. Some of the issues to consider are:

- In the United States and other Western countries, people are often "diagnosed" with ADD. People with a linear brainstyle are not assessed and diagnosed with regard to their brainstyle. In reality, people have more or fewer ADD characteristics, and the line between the "haves" and the "have-nots" is blurred.

- Many cultures would never think to identify ADD, much less diagnose it, because their worldview and behavioral style are ADD friendly. Many American Indian tribes (before the tribes were decimated by European intrusion) reflect behavior, mythology, and a lifestyle that is nonlinear in nature. The people in these settings will not be diagnosed as having a "condition."

- ADD has been primarily diagnosed in middle- and upper-class Caucasians. It is doubtful that other races and socioeconomic groups will be assessed. As one of my African American friends said, "Hey, we've got enough other things to contend with. We don't need one more thing *wrong* with us."

- The assessment of ADD can be expensive. Few low-income people have been able to access ADD assessment and service, so they are left out of the ADD count.

- People who skillfully use their ADD to advantage tend not to be "diagnosed."

- Creative people are not likely to be recognized as having ADD characteristics, though their behavior is quite similar to the traits of people considered to be ADD.

The number of people with ADD characteristics is not known. When I began work with ADD in adults in the mid-1980s, professionals claimed that from 2% to 22% of the population was affected. This large spread only began to make sense when I realized that ADD characteristics show up on a continuum rather than as a "disorder" that you have or don't have.

WHO HAS ADD?

Though this is a question frequently asked, it is only a question when the person speaking defines ADD as *something* you have or you don't have. If, as I believe, people with an ADD style of brain construction have more or fewer ADD attributes, the question no longer has meaning. It is not something you *have*, nor is it something you *are*. Rather each person has more or fewer attributes: nearly all ADD attributes, many ADD attributes, some, a few, almost none.

Possibly the spread of traits within the population of any group follows a bell-shaped curve, as many human attributes do. Maybe not. The word on the distribution of ADD traits within any population is simply not out at this time. The "Who" of ADD depends upon a number of other factors:

- Who's doing the defining of ADD and what definition of ADD are they using? Those who believe as I do will see many more people with ADD attributes than those who see ADD as a disability. Those who diagnose ADD using stringent, medical criteria will see few people as "having ADD."

Some professionals still believe ADD is a diagnosis of exclusion. This means they'll see few people who only have ADD and no coexisting "conditions." Others of us experience an ADD brainstyle as simply another dimension of human behavior. As a result, the answer to the question of "Who has ADD?" will vary greatly.

- How long does ADD last? There was a time when it was believed that only children had ADD. Then it was thought that "some children" grow into adulthood with their ADD intact. Now the majority of professionals believe ADD lasts a lifetime. Other than aging, other diversity characteristics, such as skin color, don't come and go throughout our lives. Neither does an ADD brainstyle.

- Some populations are more likely to be identified with ADD characteristics than others. Minority groups, various cultural groups, and those people living in poverty are less likely to be formally recognized or diagnosed. This could change once people worry less about diagnosing ADD and begin to accept it as a style of brain construction that is a diversity issue, not a pathological condition.

- The quieter, inwardly directed version of ADD without hyperactivity tends to be overlooked but will be present to a greater or lesser degree than other forms of ADD.

- At one time, for every female identified as ADD, there were seven males diagnosed. Professionals no longer see any difference between the rate of ADD brainstyles between males and females. Part of the explanation for the original difference may be due to the higher socialization of females. Some say it's because less pressure is placed on females to produce in linear situations.

I also wonder if the fact that girls have been observed to fit better into classroom educational settings than boys doesn't have an effect on the identification of boys as problems. And ADD has been a ready category to put these problems into. The ways in which girls express their ADD characteristics are more acceptable than boy's expressions; "cute" and "chatty," typically girls' activity, tends to be acceptable, while shooting rubber bands, typically boys' activity, is seen as disruptive.

- Those folks who have found their fit and are using ADD to advantage may not be counted.

WHY BE CONCERNED ABOUT ADD?

For each person directly affected by ADD, there are millions more—family and friends, employers, and neighbors—who experience difficulties, financially and emotionally, because of the lack of understanding of ADD attributes.

Concern 1: Stress. The high stress that people with an ADD style of brain construction suffer in a linear culture often leads to personal underachievement, frustration, and emotional discontent. In too many people, emotional health is further compromised with addictions or excesses in all forms, including eating, spending, working, and sexual acting out. Time spent in prison, often related to drug use and educational underachievement, affects a substantial number of ADD people.

Concern 2: Education. Concern about the effective education of our children brings us face-to-face with our ADD. The educational process does not tend to fit an ADD style of brain construction. In fairness, many teachers know how to teach to a diversity of brainstyles. They plan their curriculum based on sound educational principles that encompass diversity. They may or may not be supported by their school administration. But too often they are fenced in with state mandates created by noneducators or administrators who do not truly understand the meaning of diversity of brainstyles and learning processes.

The bottom line is that students with an ADD brainstyle are simply not taught in an ADD-friendly way. The time spent inefficiently trying to learn is enormous. Passing linear tests does not necessarily assess the degree to which a child or young adult has learned in school. Because the testing is skewed to linear thinkers, children may know and be able to apply the material being tested for but not be able to show what they know on a test. The time spent on teaching to the tests cheats all children of true learning, but it especially cheats ADD learners from being able to access information and thinking in the first place.

An example that devastates children in the state in which I live is the TAKS (Texas Assessment of Knowledge and Skills) test. Children spend hours being tutored so they will perform well on the test. The style of the test favors the linear learner. Unfortunately, many of those who have the biggest problem are children with ADD attributes. Not only do they have to spend more time attempting to learn how to pass the test, but also they are cheated of valuable time and opportunities to be efficiently and effectively educated.

Dropout rates are especially high in students with an ADD brainstyle. Creative, bright learners who used to do well in apprenticeship situations can no longer gain an education that fits them if they are ADD. Everyone loses as a result.

Schools lose money due to lowered test scores, and citizens' tax dollars are inefficiently used because of a failure to integrate brainstyle diversity into the education laws, mandates, and curriculum.

Concern 3: Employment. For employers, lost workdays, increased insurance rates, and low morale are other consequences of unrecognized ADD. Frequent job changes for employees who are in jobs that don't fit them cost everyone. The price of goods and services increases with employment problems, not to mention the losses to individual workers.

Promotion from a job that makes good use of an ADD style of brain to a job that requires more linear processing of information (promotion from technical/skill-based jobs to administration and supervision, for example) costs everyone. The employee loses who can't "get ahead" unless promoted to a nonfitting job. One case in point: for teachers to move up the career ladder financially, they must become administrators. Administration isn't even a first cousin to teaching. It requires totally different skills.

Concern 4: Relationships. The family of an unrecognized ADD person suffers, too. Marital conflict, expectations that cannot be fulfilled, and emotional chaos are all effects of not understanding that brainstyle diversity lives with you. Too often, couples take on the roles of parent and child, with the ADD person "performing as the child." The "parent" spouse takes on all the responsibility to manage linear tasks (such as the administration of daily living), appearing to be the responsible person in the relationship. The ADD person, already down on himself or herself, becomes more childlike and dependent, forsaking the role of "bringer of lifeblood" to the family. Often it is the zest brought by the ADD partner that captivated the heart of the linear spouse. But all those good feelings go into hiding when daily living takes over.

This is not to say if you have ADD characteristics, you can't manage a family and household. You can. But it must be done on your terms, using ADD-style approaches and problem-solving styles.

Concern about ADD needs to be a part of all of our lives. Awareness of personal ADD potential in relation to our friends, coworkers, and the community at large is essential. By each of us doing the jobs that fit our ADD style, we serve the greater good. Working as a team with our linear counterparts will bring richness to all of our lives, as diversity plays a role of creating workable solutions for our quality of life. Concerns will then disappear.

WHAT HAPPENS TO YOUR EMOTIONS WHEN YOU DISCOVER YOU HAVE AN ADD BRAINSTYLE?

When you discover you have identifiable ADD attributes, you will go through a series of stages. I first noticed this in the early 1990s at national conferences when large numbers of newly recognized ADD folks came together. They were delighted to find reasons for the experiences they had in school, in their work life, and in relationships. They were excited to find others like themselves. Eager communication followed as each shared their heartfelt feelings with others who understood, perhaps the first time ever these feelings were understood.

Watching this scene, I saw that over time the excitement and joy faded, transitioning to other feelings and behavioral expressions.

Learning to Live with ADD: Five Stages

There are five stages through which adults identified with an ADD brainstyle travel.

Stage One could be called the "Aha, I have it!" stage. "Finally, I have an explanation for why my life is the way it is. There really is *something* different about me. But I'm not crazy, retarded, lazy, inadequate, or no good."

This is a time of awakening. It's recognition that "there are others like me." "I'm not the only one." Shock, excitement, and euphoria, as well as an insatiable search for information, are likely to accompany this time.

Stage Two can be called the grief stage. Once the realization sinks in that there was a reason for not being able to live up to potential, the hurts, traumas, and losses suffered because of ADD begin to surface. As the mind begins to recall the hundreds of incidents that were related to ADD, the emotions begin to react. Confusion, anger, "what ifs," and depression all churn, creating emotional bedlam. This stage does end, but first it is important to feel the emotions and grieve the losses in order to heal the wounds.

Stage Three involves seeking support and understanding companionship during the grieving stage. This stage could be called "the family stage." Over and over at the adult ADD conferences, I heard people say, "I've found my family. There are others like me. I plan to come every year to my family reunion."

Not only can information and guidance be gained at such groupings, but all important emotional support can be obtained. "Coming home" to a place of unconditional acceptance heals the wounds of the past and supports the growth of the future.

Stage Four is characterized by seeking, exploring, and experimenting. It might be called the "growing up phase." It's a time for trying things. With ADD factored into a person's life, suddenly everything looks different. Exposure to previously tried experiences is necessary in order to discover from the new ADD perspective whether you like or dislike them, can or can't do them (especially if you use nonlinear approaches to doing them), or want or don't want to pursue them now. It's an updating of life experience data stored in your brain.

Stage Five means coming of age. It is surely a time for the unfolding of a new identity. It's a time to redefine values, honor talents and gifts, and love who and what you are. "I know who I am now. I believe in myself. I can do whatever I've discovered I like. I am me." Reaching potential is wonderful, beautiful, and heady stuff. It is also possible and real.

The integration of current information into the life experiences of innumerable people is opening the door for the development of a valuable resource known to each of us: individual identity. As differences are recognized and diversity of brainstyles is honored, not only will individuals' lives be made more pleasant, but also the world will truly become a better place in which to live.

Let us provide support through the five stages of healing and growth of those with ADD in a context of understanding and acceptance. Let us provide mentorship. Let us take responsibility to spread the word that ADD is a normal, wonderful style of brain construction that reflects another dimension of human diversity. Let us stand up and refuse to be called disordered, handicapped, deficit, or in any way abnormal. In this way, everyone wins.

I've written this book in an ADD-friendly way using stories, personal experiences, and phrases in the text that reflect an ADD perspective more than a linear one. As one who draws primarily from hands-on field experiences rather than an in-house research environment, however, I want to be sure to include current research done in laboratories using the scientific method. I've asked John Rubel to summarize the current findings available from such research.

ADD RESEARCH UPDATE, BY JOHN RUBEL, PSY.D.

Imperfect Lenses

Try as they might, researchers and clinicians who investigate ADD (the authors included) aren't perfectly objective. In attempting to synthesize a body of data, we arrive at some synthetic judgment that has been contaminated by our theory-driven confirmatory biases, motivated distortions, and other sources of error (Kuhn, 1962).

Yet our clinical judgment, albeit flawed, is essential for identifying potentially relevant variables and patterns, framing hypotheses, and building theories about ADD (Westen & Weinberger, 2004).

The evolving optics of Dr. Weiss's and my struggle to synthesize our experiences of the tension between the current state of ADD science and clinical practice is called "brainstyle theory." Before presenting our theory, let's briefly review the scientific research on ADD.

Overview of the Research Big Picture

1. The overwhelming majority of individuals with ADD have no history of significant brain injuries (Barkley, 1998).

2. Neuropsychological testing of ADD individuals has detected some differences in frontal lobe functions, but those findings are inconsistent (Barkley, 1997).

3. Researchers have been unable to document with any certainty neurochemical or neurotransmitter deficiencies as causal factors for ADD (Barkley, 1998).

4. Nervous system psychophysiological measures have been inconsistent in demonstrating significant group differences between ADD individuals and controls (Baumeister & Hawkins, 2001).

5. ADD neuro-imaging studies have not found evidence for any type of brain structural damage (Leo & Cohen, 2002; Overmeyer & Taylor, 2001; Frank & Pavlakis, 2001).

6. There is no compelling evidence that pregnancy or birth complications cause ADD (Barkley, 1998).

7. Due to serious methodological limitations, the evidence that ADD is caused by environmental toxins, for example, prenatal exposure to alcohol and tobacco smoke or elevated body lead levels, must be viewed with caution (Barkley, 1998).

8. No evidence exists to show that ADD is the result of abnormal, damaged, or extra chromosomes. There is convincing evidence of a family hereditary basis or genetic link for ADD (Biederman et al., 1995; Faraone, 2000).

9. Although the present technology of neuro-imaging studies may help determine the volume and shape of brain structures involved in a specific cognitive task, they cannot provide information about the timing and rapid order of neuronal firing, nor can they show the oscillations between cortical and subcortical brain networks that are hypothesized to bind and integrate neural systems (Durston et al., 2001; Stern & Silbersweig, 2001).

Interpretation

Although peer-reviewed scientific research has discovered many neurobiological correlations associated with ADD, there is no solid, conclusive evidence about the cause(s) of ADD, or that ADD brains are dysfunctional, damaged, or deficient. Perhaps ADD brains are diverse and different.

Brainstyle: Right or Wrong? Good or Bad? Or ? A friend asks you to help her. She has purchased a life-size mechanical dog robot for her son's birthday, and she needs you to assemble it. You put the large box in your car, drive home, and carry it into your living room. What do you do next?

If your brainstlye is similar to mine, you will proceed more or less as follows:

1. Before opening the box, lay out *all* the tools you anticipate needing.
2. Carefully open the box, remove *only* the assembly instructions, and read over them several times.
3. Cautiously remove the box's contents, looking over each part and checking it against the assembly diagram.
4. Arrange the parts in the order you will need them.
5. Begin the assembly at step one, and *only* proceed to step two after you have checked and rechecked your work.
6. Several hours, or days, later, push the on button, give thanks that you've finished, and pray the dog will bark and wag its tail. If not, consider taking a mood stabilizer medication and start all over.

If your brainstyle is similar to Lynn's, you will behave as follows:

1. You will glance at the pictures on the box, making a mental image of what the assembled dog robot will look like.

2. Drawing on your past experiences of assembling similar mechanical objects, you will start to intuitively feel what you need to do.

3. You will open the box, dump out all its contents, and start putting the robot together. You will pay little attention to the detailed instructions except for an occasional glance at a pictorial diagram that you may find helpful.

4. After the assembly is completed, you will push the "on" button. If the robot dog fails to bark and wag its tail, you will tinker with it until it works, or until your frustration level renders you temporarily helpless.

So, which way is better? According to brainstyle theory, the answer is neither. Both brainstyles have their advantages and disadvantages, depending on the situational context. Brainstyles, like our skin color, gender, sexual orientation, religion, and culture, are another facet of human diversity, albeit a largely invisible one.

What Are Brainstyles and Where Do They Come From? Visualize your brainstyle as a three-sided pyramid filled with energy that can be readily transferred throughout its structure. The base of your pyramid comprises neurons and neural networks that predispose you to develop certain biological, cognitive, and temperamental traits (Tyron, 2002; Cloniger et al., 1993). The structure and function of your neural network base is influenced by the genes you inherited and, more importantly, your developmental learning.

One side of your brainstyle pyramid consists of what psychologists call cognitive information-processing mechanisms, such as attention and memory. We all exhibit different abilities in these areas (Fernandez-Duque & Posner, 2001). For example, some brainstyles readily attend to auditory stimuli, whereas others prefer visual stimuli. The working memory of brainstyles may be organized around cognitive data or kinesthetic data. Recent research suggests that cognitive information-processing mechanisms are trainable, especially in young children (Murray, 2003).

Your motivational system and characteristic manner of behaving comprises the second side of your brainstyle pyramid (Sternberg & Grisorenko, 1997). Some people prefer highly structured situations with explicit rules while others perform best in unstructured situations that have minimal restrictions. Some people enjoy completing one task at a time while others prefer working on multiple tasks simultaneously. Some people prefer routine and familiarity in life whereas others crave novelty and change.

The third side of your brainstyle pyramid is the environment in which you live (Kuo & Faber Taylor, 2004). If your environment is a reasonably "good fit" for your neural network, cognitive information-processing mechanisms, and motivational system/characteristic manner of behavior, then your chances for success and fulfillment are quite good.

But what if it's a "bad fit?" What if your primary caretakers, teachers, and significant others have a different brainstyle than you and, as a consequence, judge your brainstyle to be defective? What if you repeatedly find yourself failing in situations designed for other types of brainstyles (Galves et al., 2004)? The what ifs could go on forever, but the end result of environmental invalidation is low self-esteem, increased emotional dis-ease, and a tendency to either behaviorally withdraw or act out.

Conversely, what if you grew up in an environment that understood, valued, and supported the natural attributes of different brainstyles? The end result on individuals and society as a whole would be very different.

Brainstyle theory hypothesizes that, like many other human characteristics, brainstyles are normally distributed. One half of the distribution is represented by linear (non-ADD) brainstyles such as mine, the other half by nonlinear (ADD) brainstyles such as Lynn's. Individuals whose brainstyles fall near the end of either side of the distribution are likely to encounter more environment situations that are a "bad fit."

In the past, these people have been labeled as having a mental disorder. There is no denying the personal suffering these individuals experience. However, brainstyle theory proposes this suffering can be eliminated if individuals choose:

1. to recognize and understand their unique brainstyle attributes;
2. to assertively educate others about brainstyle diversity;
3. to select environments that are a better fit for their brainstyle; and
4. to develop compensatory strategies and skills that supplement the natural tendencies of their brainstyle.

In summary, brainstyles are a construct encompassing the unique neurobiological, cognitive, social-behavioral, and environmental aspects of each individual. Each side of the brainstyle pyramid, including the base, is influenced by what happens to every other side. Although this may sound deceivingly simple, in reality it is exceedingly complex. Advances in scientific imaging technologies and interdisciplinary fields of research, referred to as social cognitive neuroscience (Ochsner & Lieberman, 2001), have just begun to explore these reciprocal interconnections.

Dr. Rubel's research update supports the position proposed in this book. In 2002, through his membership in the Division of Psychotherapy (Division 29) of the American Psychological Association, Dr. Rubel received a copy of their brochure on Attention Deficit–Hyperactivity Disorder. He became aware of a response written by Al Galves, Ph.D., a Colorado psychologist, in response to the same brochure. Rubel recently spoke with Dr. Galves and opened the doorway for me to dialogues with Galves about his dialogue with Division 29.

In 2002, Al Galves entered into a dialogue with the Division of Psychotherapy (Division 29) of the American Psychological Association regarding a brochure the division published on Attention Deficit–Hyperactivity Disorder. Displeased with the content of the brochure, Galves wrote to Dr. Alice Rubenstein, the director of the Brochure Project, expressing his concern. I asked Galves to summarize what happened as a result.

DIALOGUE REGARDING ADD RESEARCH DIVISION 29 OF THE AMERICAN PSYCHOLOGICAL ASSOCIATION, BY AL GALVES, PH.D.

In early 2002, I received a copy of a brochure on Attention Deficit–Hyperactivity Disorder (ADHD) that had been published and distributed by the Division of Psychotherapy (Division 29) of the American Psychological Association. Aware that ADHD was a lynchpin in the movement to portray mental illness as a result of random biological forces, I reviewed the brochure carefully for evidence of that ideology. I was especially careful in view of the fact that the brochure had been financed by Celltech Pharmaceuticals, which manufacturers and distributes methylphenidate, the most popular drug used to treat ADHD.

Sure enough, I found the following three statements that support the ideology of biopsychiatry but are not supported by adequate scientific evidence:

1. "ADD/ADHD is generally considered a neuro-chemical disorder."

2. "Most people with ADD/ADHD are born with the disorder, though it may not be recognized until adulthood."

3. "ADHD is not caused by poor parenting, a difficult family environment, poor teaching or inadequate nutrition."

My reaction was a combination of outrage and despair. Here was the Division of Psychotherapy, presumably comprising psychologists least in the thrall of pharmaceutical companies, falling prey to the ideology of biopsychiatry and getting into bed with the drug companies. Here was a group of professionals who prided themselves on being scientist-practitioners endorsing statements that were not backed by adequate scientific evidence. And, apparently, I was the only one of the 4,000 members of the division who was concerned about it.

I wrote a letter to Dr. Alice Rubenstein, director of the Brochure Project, expressing concern about the statements. Dr. Rubenstein wrote back telling me that she had shared my letter with Dr. Robert Resnick, under whose presidency the Brochure Project had been initiated, and Dr. Kalman Heller, a member of Division 29. In the letter, Dr. Rubenstein included references to back up the statement that "evidence to date suggests a biological cause."

I spent the better part of a year studying the references that had been supplied by Drs. Resnick and Heller and looking at other scientific evidence on the forces and factors that contribute to the behavior that results in children being diagnosed with ADHD.

With the help of Dr. David Walker, a fellow member of Division 29, I sent a 24-page letter back to Dr. Rubenstein. The letter clearly demonstrated that there is as much, if not more, evidence refuting the statements in the brochure as there is supporting it, thereby exposing the three statements as ideology masquerading as fact.

I found that the evidence used to support the statement that ADHD is a neurochemical disorder is flawed in two major ways. First, the research demonstrating a difference between the brains of children diagnosed with ADHD and those not so diagnosed failed to control for the fact that the great majority of the subjects with ADHD had been taking psychostimulant drugs (Ritalin) for years prior to the research and the possibility that the drugs were the cause of the brain differences.

Second, even if the evidence were not contaminated by that research flaw, a difference in the brains of the children would not be evidence that ADHD is a neurochemical disorder. To think so is to confuse correlation with causation. If, in fact, the brains of children diagnosed with ADHD are significantly different from those of persons not so diagnosed, it is more likely that such brain differences are a *result* of psychological variables such as thoughts, feelings, habits, assumptions, beliefs, and intentions than a *cause* of them. After all, that is the case with the mind-body dynamic that has been most thoroughly subjected to scientific investigation: the stress response. In the stress response, a profound physiological response is *preceded* by the perception of threat and cognitive awareness that it is real and requires a response.

There is lots of evidence that supports the probability that changes in brain physiology are the results rather than the cause of thoughts, feelings, and intentions. Here are two examples:

Jeffrey Schwartz investigated the impact of both psychotropic drugs and cognitive-behavioral (talk) therapy on the brains of patients diagnosed with Obsessive-Compulsive Disorder. He found that the drugs and the talk therapy had the same impact on brain physiology.

Researchers at Cornell University found that the brains of children who had trouble reading were different from those of good readers. After providing the poor readers with intensive instruction in reading, they found that not only were the children reading better, but also that their brain physiology had changed.

The point here is that we don't have the scientific capability to tease out the causal relationships between psychological and biological variables. So people—even people who pride themselves on being scientists—believe what they want to believe. Certainly, there is not enough scientific evidence to support the statement that was made in the Division 29 brochure.

I found that the evidence that supports the belief that people are born with ADHD—that it is a result of genetic determinism—is equally flawed. The studies that were cited by Drs. Resnick and Heller base their conclusion on the fact that interclass correlations for the symptoms of ADHD are significantly greater between monozygotic than between dizygotic twins. In order to impute a genetic explanation for this finding, it must be assumed that monozygotic and dizygotic twins grow up in equal environments. But such is not the case. Research has demonstrated that monozygotic twins spend more time together, study together more, have the same close friends, attend the same social events, are more closely attached, are more inseparable as children, experience more identity confusion in childhood, and are emotionally closer than dizygotic twins. The research also fails to describe how gene expression might influence the kind of behavior that is used to diagnose ADHD and fails to account for the complexity of gene expression, a process involving the synthesis of proteins that would presumably be influenced by environmental factors.

Finally and most importantly, the research fails to account for the impact of the mother-infant bond during the first year of life on the later behavior of children. The simple fact is that not since John Bowlby and Mary Ainsworth did their seminal research on the attachment between mother and infant have any researchers been present to observe the interaction between mother and infant during the first year of life. In the absence of reliable data about those interactions and their impact on the later behavior of children, no evidence of genetic determinism is believable.

I found that the evidence that "ADHD is not caused by poor parenting, a difficult family environment, poor teaching or inadequate nutrition" is contaminated by a similar failure to adequately account for the potential influence of all of those factors on the behavior of children. In fact, a preponderance of evidence has found that the behavior associated with ADHD is significantly associated with unmet needs for nurturance in childhood, difficult family environments, and inhumane and oppressive school and community environments. To cite one example, Alfie Cohn noted that children whose behavior in today's rigidly structured classrooms leads to ADHD diagnoses don't behave that way in open classrooms, leading him to question whether we are diagnosing children or classroom environments.

In my letter to Dr. Rubenstein, I explained that my concern over the false statements was not academic. My main concern was that the statements reflect the ideology of biopsychiatry that supports treatment regimens that are harmful to children. Harmful because giving children drugs fails to honor their behavior as a functional response to a situation that for them is difficult, off-putting, oppressive, discounting, boring, and/or irrelevant. Harmful because it fails to use the child's crisis as an opportunity for learning how to manage emotions, thoughts, intentions, and behavior in more adaptive and life-enhancing ways rather than as an opportunity to learn how to use drugs. Harmful because the drugs have damaging side effects that have yet to be adequately subjected to scientific investigation. Harmful, finally, because the ideology of biopsychiatry makes it easier to do nothing about improving the school, family, and community environments that are so damaging to some children.

In our letter to Dr. Rubenstein, which was cosigned by 10 other members of Division 29, Walker and I asked the division to cease distribution of the brochures and to produce another brochure that "reflects a more balanced account of the available scientific evidence and the wide diversity of views of practicing psychologists regarding ADHD."

To date, Division 29 has not responded in any material way to the letter. This experience opened my eyes to the amazing influence that the ideology of biopsychiatry has had on psychologists in this country. It makes me wonder about the future of psychology and psychotherapy.

4

THE QUANDARY OF "TREATMENT"

Sherry originally came into therapy wanting help with her second marriage. She was angry at her husband because he didn't take enough financial responsibility, and the children (his and hers) were erupting right and left. There were individual motivations, too. Her mood swings, evident all her life, seemed to be growing more extreme. Her ability to focus on a task and complete it seemed to have diminished rather than to have grown.

But she seemed eager to get things right in her life, ready to work at therapy. The only problem to the upbeat beginning was that Sherry had a different agenda every time she came in for therapy. Every time she agreed to work on an issue, something got in the way and follow-through was avoided. She would go off in a dozen directions the minute she walked out of my office.

Sherry's husband, though not as scattered, was no better than she was at follow-through. He made even bigger promises that he didn't keep. When he drank, he became playful and less responsible than when he was sober. He'd grin sheepishly when confronted about his behavior. Working with the two of them turned out to be next to impossible.

Going through problems with each of their five children as the teenage years arrived, Sherry and her husband were not able to take charge. They knew what to do but couldn't implement what they had planned.

Then the husband's financial irresponsibility left them in a lot of trouble, which Sherry felt helpless to remedy. And Sherry, who for years had worked with her father (a drinker who had encouraged dependence in Sherry), was left without a job when he retired; the secure, if damaging, daily routine that had put structure in her life was eliminated.

Her husband's response was to face the music (his accountant and the IRS) and clean up his act. He stopped drinking, shaped up physically, and began to take responsibility in his business.

But it wasn't long after that that Sherry began drinking heavily and abusing her body in other ways—binging on caffeine products and eating and sleeping erratically. Eventually, she became bulimic. Then other self-destructive behaviors began to emerge. Sherry started to act out her feelings, which meant, in her words, "pulling a runaway." She'd simply leave home, taking up with whomever she met. Maybe she'd have an affair, maybe just a friendship punctuated by raucous emotional highs.

She'd claim great insights into her psychology from these episodes, but her scattered behavior didn't change, nor did her life smooth out. Much of the acting out was met with passivity by her husband, while her father supplied financial support so that Sherry could remain irresponsible. She continued being out of control for almost two years, until she became an excessive financial liability and her mood swings (days spent in bed intermixed with days on the run) had increased to the point where they could no longer be ignored. She was hospitalized four times during that next year.

Professionals who worked with Sherry disagreed about what was *wrong* with her. Their diagnoses ranged from alcoholism to Attention Deficit Disorder, manic depression characterized by wide mood swings, and borderline personality characterized by a pervasive pattern of instability. A few more diagnoses were thrown in for good measure.

Maybe they were all correct, for Sherry was a classic example of a person displaying multiple disorders, or at least the symptoms of such. Her childhood history—at school and in the family—indicated that she certainly had an ADD-style brain. Her mother had died when she was five. From that time on, she was raised by a dysfunctional family that was riddled by addiction and codependency. Sherry never properly separated from her family of origin to become an independent grown-up with value in her own right.

She lived at a survival level most of the time, just barely able to show enough responsibility to get by. Her biochemistry was out of balance, in part because she did not attend to her nutrition, exercise, and rest. Her mood swings, from extreme emotional highs to severe depression, were separated by periods of mood normality that occurred when she worked for her father in a highly structured job.

An extreme case? You bet, but Sherry's situation points out how difficult it can be to make a proper identification of an

ADD brainstyle when it's buried under clinical disorders and symptoms that overlap.

ADD is not a "diagnosis" of exclusion any more than skin color. It can coexist with other emotional and neurological issues. All the characteristics of ADD can also be seen in learning disabilities. Mood variability can be the result of hormones, nutritional inadequacy, and stress, and/or a part of ADD sensitivity, when a person reacts to what is happening in his or her environment. Impulsivity and overreactivity can be the result of poor or inadequate training or other organic difficulties, including seizure disorders. It can also occur when a person is placed in a highly frustrating environment that doesn't fit.

To further complicate the problem, mimicking symptoms may be present: stress and emotional difficulties can mimic many ADD characteristics, such as inattentiveness to detail, low self-esteem, and anger. But being ADD is neither abnormal nor symptomatic, unless the diagnostician *judges* one brainstyle to be abnormal in relation to another. Being moody, inattentive, and impulsive because of a head injury or as the result of emotional trauma, post-traumatic stress disorder (PTSD), and childhood abuse is more likely to be judged pathological.

When we consider Sherry's choices, the picture becomes cloudier. As if whipped around at the end of a tether line, Sherry's choices changed from moment to moment as her varying "problems" took the forefront. To deal effectively with her ADD, she would have had to isolate her brainstyle's functioning from the morass of other clinical issues.

After I referred Sherry for addiction counseling, she was pushed too hard by her new therapist. Her ADD sensitivity further enlarged the effects of his confrontations, leaving her unable to retain the gains she'd made in previous counseling. When the clinician moved too fast and harshly with her right at the time she was steadily, for the first time, building a sense of her own inner power and control, she was thrown back into a victim role, from which she did not recover. This occurred following successful hypnotherapy to reframe some of her childhood trauma. It preceded the beginning of her "runaways" and subsequent total breakdown.

Making choices builds emotional powerfulness. But when a fledgling new self is emerging, delicacy, restraint, and firm support are needed to protect the emerging self. In situations where alcohol abuse is present, firm insistence on the cessation of drinking is imperative. There's a fine line between firmness and harshness when dealing with addiction and ADD at the same time. Firm support of the emerging True Self becomes essential to protect any budding powerfulness in the person.

This discussion of potential responses to Attention Deficit Disorder is based on the assumption that ADD is a perfectly normal way to be constructed. It is important to differentiate the normalcy of your innate brainstyle from conditions that are the result of some causative factor that creates look-alike symptoms.

For example, inattention to details by a nonlinear person is natural when the details are lined up in a row one after the other. Details that are a part of a process, part of a flow, or the creation of feelings can be worked with by someone with an ADD-style brain. The ADD person simply looks at the big picture and steadily extracts the details as needed. Thus inattention to details that are linear in nature is no more abnormal for someone with a lot of ADD characteristics than inattention to details that are nonlinear in nature is abnormal for someone who primarily has a linear brainstyle. But inattention to all details, no matter what the brainstyle or the setting, would be considered abnormal.

You will want to assess informally or formally the likelihood of your having ADD attributes. You can do this by filling out a checklist, listening to a presentation that reflects the way you are, or going to a clinician who specializes in the assessment of ADD. You will want to separate your ADD brainstyle traits from others that are a reflection of physical or mental problems and addictions.

This does not need to be done in minute detail. But do recognize that many people, regardless of brainstyle, have "issues" to deal with. Do not fall into the trap of blaming all your problems on ADD. You can work on both adjusting to your ADD brainstyle at the same time you work with other self-improvement skills.

Once you've figured out that you have an ADD brainstyle and you want to maximize your effective use of the True You (the unfettered way in which you are constructed), you have choices and decisions to make about how to proceed.

YOUR QUANDARY

The quandary you face as someone with an ADD brainstyle comes in relation to the question, "What shall I do about how I am constructed?"

There is a need to help you to learn skills that can make use of your ADD brainstyle. These are nonlinear methods of organization, behavioral and emotional expression. You can achieve any skill in a non-linear way that you wish to develop. The True You can then emerge to your satisfaction.

The hurt and pain suffered because of being exposed to situations and expectations that don't fit you must be treated to heal the Wounded You. Trauma reduction, emotional power building, and relief from the symptoms of pain and suffering all must be attended to. Emergence from your wounded past must be achieved while keeping your ADD sensitivity in mind, if good results are to be expected.

There is also a need to help you and all people with a predominantly ADD brainstyle to survive linear situations. When confronting situations that don't fit you, your Accommodating Self faces a challenge and you must ask yourself what you want to do about it.

The needs of the Accommodating Self are different from those of the Wounded Self. Instead of treatment, the Accommodating Self requires specially designed *training* for you to function successfully in environments that don't readily fit you but in which you need to function to achieve the goals you desire. You must, however, remember that there is nothing inherently wrong with *you*, just with a situation in which you find yourself.

Typical challenges that you will have to face:

- You may be in a situation such as school in which your normal style cannot get the grades you need or want. You simply are not able to use your strengths effectively. Or you may be forced to continually work from a position of weakness.

- You may *have* to use linear skills to accomplish a goal you desire.

- For the time being, you may have to "fake it 'til you make it." Perhaps you do not yet have the power or authority to

> do things in a way that fits you. So you must pretend to be something you're not until you acquire the experience that will promote you to a position of power. Then you can do things as you wish as long as you accomplish the goal in a timely manner.

Let's consider the two categories of options available to you—treatment and training—to counteract the challenges you face.

TREATMENT AND TRAINING

Treatment brings with it the idea that there is something *wrong* with you and it needs to be made well. Therefore, treatment is relegated to helping with the healing of the Wounded You, not the True You. It's fine for you to "be treated," as long as you keep in mind the point that there is nothing inherently wrong with you. You don't have to remake yourself. You don't have to change yourself permanently for all situations.

Instead, I would suggest that you think of treatment as a short-term solution to assist you to move into a lifestyle that honors your natural strengths. It will also help you heal the Wounded You so you won't be distracted from living as fully as the True You is designed to live. In most cases, treatment can also be used for a short period of time while you are training the Accommodating You.

Training does not attempt to alter your innate brainstyle, but instead to make it work more effectively for you. You build up your mental muscle to achieve tasks in ways that fit you. You can go after any goal that is generally thought to be important, but you must do it in a way that uses your strengths.

For example, organizing paper (or anything else) so you can find it is a goal. Putting the papers in a file cabinet by alphabetical order with name labels attached is a linear way to organize. Putting the papers in color-coded stacks by project or function is a nonlinear way to organize them. Both serve the same purpose. Neither is right or wrong. Each is just a different way of accomplishing the goal.

As an ADD person, I know you will have your own creative, individualistic ways to accomplish tasks. You can observe yourself while paying attention to what you do and how you naturally do it, and you'll learn from your observations what works for you. Or you can use a mentor or guidelines discovered by someone else to help you find what works for you (see *The New Attention Deficit Disorder in Adults Workbook*). In the end, you'll build a system that is your own. Therefore, it will bring you success.

TREATING ADD

Let's look at treatment options that are available to you. We'll begin with the use of prescription medication to assist you to fit into mismatching situations or to buy you the time to learn new living skills. Also, I'll cover the "treatment" of abuse and inner pain that is the result of your having been inappropriately handled. Finally, you'll see the virtue of using groups to heal your hurts and give you new hope and the motivation to seek training.

A traditional resource for treating ADD is the prescribing of medications. To this end, Keith Caramelli, M.D., a practicing psychiatrist in Austin, Texas, agreed to be interviewed for this fourth edition. He is trained in both pediatric and adult psychiatry. He currently maintains a private practice in addition to participating in a multispecialty group practice with Austin Child Guidance Center and the Oaks Treatment Center in Austin.

Medication and ADD: An Interview with Keith Caramelli, M.D.

LW: How did you become interested in Attention Deficit Disorder?

KC: My interest largely evolved out of the large population of children that present to me as a child psychiatrist with concerns from the school and parents about the disorder. I think the condition took on greater interest to me when I became aware that the stimulant medications used to treat ADD improve concentration, decrease impulsivity, and decrease distractibility in children without ADD symptoms as well as those with the condition.

LW: What is most important to consider when talking about medicating adults?

KC: Most important would be evaluating the level of impairment that the attentional symptoms are causing the patient. These obviously need to be weighed against the drawbacks of taking a psychotropic medication. A history of substance abuse is also very important to consider when evaluating the use of stimulant medications.

LW: What about self-diagnosis and a medication request?

KC: In general, I am leery of self-diagnosis. I would expect that the individual would have some tangible collateral information from work and/or family that illustrated the extent of impairment in functioning. I guess when we are talking about a request for medication I would expect that the individual had explored other learning or behavioral methods to accommodate his/her attentional problems before seeking medicine.

LW: Under what conditions do you consider recommending medication for adults who have the ADD style of brain construction? Who are good candidates?

KC: I think the first thing to consider is the true extent of impairment of functioning in multiple areas of the individual's life. I would expect the individual to have a history of impairment dating back to school days. Again, I think a good candidate would be someone who has invested himself into finding ways to adapt to the way their brain learns prior to seeking a pharmacological solution.

LW: What drugs do you consider using for the treatment of ADD in adults?

KC: Really, all drugs that are utilized in children for ADHD are worth utilizing in adults. This includes the stimulants (methylphenidate, amphetamine sulphate, dextroamphetamine), antidepressants (buproprion and possibly others), and atomoxetine.

LW: How does a physician know what medications to choose?

KC: To a large extent this has to do with matching the side effects with the individual. For instance, patients with a substance abuse history are probably not good candidates for the stimulants, which are controlled substances. Stimulants have the advantage that they are effective within approximately one hour after taking them and are worn off and out of the system within 12 hours. This type of pharmacological action would allow an individual to take the medication on the day that he or she knew that it would be needed and not on other days, such as the weekend, etc.

Alternately, atomoxetine, which is a nonstimulant ADD agent, probably takes at least five days before it begins demonstrating a significant therapeutic effect. Further, this medication would be expected to work best when a consistent level was maintained in the blood so irregular usage would not be recommended. Unlike stimulants, however, a single dose of atomoxetine is believed to last greater than 24 hours so individuals who have difficulties with the stimulant medication wearing off may do better with an agent such as atomoxetine. Lastly, buproprion may not be as powerful in effecting concentration changes. However, it works independently on depressive symptoms which may be indicated in individuals who have comorbid depressive symptoms.

LW: What are indicators that the medication is working?

KC: I look for the patient expressing an improved ability to concentrate on a task, improved ability to stick with a task that was previously difficult to complete, a self-observed ability to be more organized and typically less frustrated and overwhelmed. In general, I would expect some corroboration of these changes by others interacting with the individual whether it be a partner in the relationship or coworker on the job.

LW: What are indicators that the medication is not working?

KC: Generally, no observed effect. In truth, if there is no observed effect to the patient on a stimulant medication, I have to reevaluate whether I am treating the correct diagnosis.

LW: How long might a person expect to take ADD medications? And what about "Use as Needed"?

KC: There are some individuals who I believe may use medication throughout much of their life. I believe this would be the extreme minority. In general, I believe that in adulthood, most people can develop adequate coping tools to manage effectively without medication through most of their lives. That said, I do believe that there is a case to be made for the use of the medications as needed for special situations.

LW: Speak to the issue of dual diagnosis.

KC: My first thought as a psychiatrist is to treat the other psychiatric diagnosis first and evaluate whether there is any improvement in the attention symptoms as a consequence of improvement of the primary psychiatric diagnosis. Sometimes, both conditions can be treated at the same time, as in the case when a depressed individual with ADD responds to the antidepressant Welbutrin. Other times, the primary psychiatric condition can make treatment of ADD more difficult, as is the case when an anxiety disorder is worsened by stimulant medication or buproprion. Sometimes, the psychiatric condition is a consequence of the frustration from the difficulties in dealing with the symptoms of ADD and can improve rapidly with the appropriate behavioral or medication treatment of ADD.

LW: If a person has a history of drug or alcohol abuse, what are your thoughts regarding use of medication?

KC: I would probably be reluctant to use the stimulant medications (which are controlled substances) in individuals with histories of substance abuse. That said, every patient is an individual, and I would take the individual's personal history and recovery into close consideration. Additionally, most stimulants are prescribed in long-acting preparations now which make the misuse of the medicine for abuse purposes more difficult.

LW: In addition to medication, what else do you feel people with ADD need in order to better live up to their potential?

KC: Most importantly, I think everyone needs a support system. This means other people who have some understanding of the difficulties that ADD can create in day-to-day life and an interest in understanding and supporting the individual struggling with this problem. I believe everyone needs encouragement and can benefit from guidance to help them maximize their own individual assets.

LW: What else would you like people to know about ADD?

KC: I suspect that I don't perceive this "diagnosis" as disabling as many do. I do believe that there are assets that accompany the symptoms of ADD that may be quite valuable but are not valued enough. I believe that a majority of adult individuals who can fulfill a diagnosis of ADD can develop coping mechanisms which will serve them better than medications in the long run.

See appendix C for a chart of commonly used medications with the name of the manufacturers, generic names, attributes, and other pertinent information.

Grief

The need to treat grief is common with people who have an ADD brainstyle. Fortunately, such treatment is well documented, effective, and easy to access.

Grief is a normal reaction to loss of any kind, including self-esteem and your dreams. Because of your ADD style of brain construction, you may have given up on your dreams because you didn't see a way of achieving them. Then there's the loss of potential in general. There may be tangible losses, too, such as the loss of a marriage, relationships, jobs, or educational opportunities. All of these leave feelings of grief. That's normal.

Know that you can learn about and overcome the first four stages of grief—denial, anger, bargaining or guilt, and depression—until you are able to achieve acceptance or change, which is the fifth stage. Then you can start over with the new you who believes in yourself so the True You can have a fresh start.

You can often work at the healing of your grief yourself. Or you may wish to seek the help of others who are like you. They can provide you with support and may mentor you through the grief process. A peer group works well for this purpose.

Finally, if your feelings are too raw or too big to be managed by yourself or in a setting with peers, consider seeking counseling. Give yourself permission to reach out for professional help to get over the initial hump blocking your way to recovery from the ravages of your grief.

If you choose to work on your own or in a peer group, here are some things you can do. Take what fits or feels okay to you and set aside what doesn't.

- Commit to getting the training you need to function effectively with your ADD brainstyle. (See *The New Attention Deficit Disorder in Adults Workbook.*)

- If you prefer to go it alone, fine. You may be your own best counsel.

- Come together with anyone who will be a good listener and give you support: a friend, relative, or spiritual or religious confidant.

- Come together with others who are in the same situation you are.

- Identify where you are in the grief process. You may be feeling more than one of these at a time or experiencing the feelings in a different order:

    - Denial—"I can't believe there's a reason I've done so poorly. I've just always been a 'klutz.' It's the way I am."

  - Anger—“It’s the fault of the system. It’s not fair that I was treated the way I was.”
  - Guilt—“I should have worked harder.”
  - Depression—“It’s hopeless. I’m too old to change.”
  - Acceptance—“I’m fine the way I am. I’ll let go of what I lost before and consider what I want to go after now.”

- If you like the idea of sharing with a group, express the feelings you have one at a time, but avoid repeating them over and over. This expression can take the form of storytelling. Everyone has a story, and telling that story will show you and others that none of us is alone.

- Consider rewriting your life story with a new ending. Journaling can be a big help with this, besides being fulfilling for you. You can journal or talk about what you would change about what happened to you at an earlier time. Then in your mind’s eye, see that change happening. This can be done alone or in a group activity in which everyone has suggestions. What a great way to feel supported!

- Let yourself dream of the way or ways in which the new you would like to live and be expressive: on the job, with your family, in your life, and personally.

- Set small goals to acquire the skills you need to make your dreams real.

- Ask for help from your group members, friends, or family who are supportive when you run into a hitch. Get some suggestions for how to get beyond the problem and use only ones that *feel* right to you.

- If drug or alcohol use is involved, immediately get into treatment. You can do ADD training at the same time, or you may learn about handling your ADD after you are in recovery.

- Consider using your feelings creatively. You may be drawn to write stories or plays or make paintings that first express your hurt feelings and then your transformed, healed feelings.

Specialized Treatment of Anger, Flooding, Confusion, and Impulsivity

Anger can be reframed by understanding what its role is and then finding other ways to use the energy. Anger is always present to help protect your vulnerable feelings from too much hurt and pain. That's a worthy cause. But too often, anger takes on a life of its own. When that happens, you don't get what you really want and neither does anyone else. In fact, chaos is more likely to be the outcome.

Your anger is like a shield; there is a time and place to raise it protectively. In order to heal, you must make a choice about whether to use your anger as a shield or as a controlled action to make a difference in the world. It is a message to be understood. Understanding this, and acting accordingly, is necessary if you are to heal. Here are the steps you can take in order to make your anger constructive:

- Move to a safe place where you can look at the feelings and motivations beneath your shield of anger.

- Be supported or shielded by others or your own strength before you peek at what lies beneath your anger. You will find one or more of the following: fear, frustration, feelings of helplessness, and feelings of hopelessness.

- Once you've found what lies beneath your anger, begin to problem solve solutions for what is bothering you. You may find it extremely helpful to ask others who you sense have been down the path ahead of you. You may choose to go within yourself and meditate or do other inner work that you've learned to rely upon.

- See yourself as capable of being self-protective in situations that previously have caused you problems.

- Resolve to walk away from or avoid situations that are harmful and that show no signs of changing. If another person is involved, determine whether or not the person can go halfway, taking half of the responsibility for the problem. If not, you must work alone and fix yourself. Then decide how you want to relate to the person.

- Use your anger constructively to make lasting changes where you see wrong rather than blowing up in the short term.

Flooding is the condition where too much stimulation and input come your way, getting through your defenses. Being sensitive, you may not have strong, thick boundaries, emotionally speaking, to fend off external stimuli. Most commonly, shopping malls, huge crowds, tightly packed rooms, and lots of stimulating goings-on are the culprits in a flooding event. There's just too much energy circulating, and since we pick up things the average person doesn't, we absorb all that energy and it overloads our circuits.

We tend to absorb the energy of the people around us. Frenzy, anxiety, out-of-control behavior, and fear all cross our sensitive boundaries so we feel what belongs to another person.

This capacity was useful when I was a diagnostician, but it sure isn't something I want to have to deal with in my daily living. I also don't want to have to keep my guard up all the time.

The sensation of flooding is confusing and threatening. Don't be surprised if you react with feelings of desperation or even have an anxiety attack. Lessening the pain of anxiety, though certainly a humane response, doesn't get to the core of the problem. Rather, you'll benefit long term by learning to manage your ADD sensitivity that leads to flooding.

For the short term, shut your eyes, lean on something, or better yet, someone, remember to breathe evenly and moderately, visualize a calm, peaceful setting in your mind, and slowly remove yourself from the overstimulating environment. In the long run, simply remember to avoid such settings. I, for one, don't shop during rush hour and don't like big crowds or entertainment venues that are tightly packed. There's just too much wild energy moving around for me to deal with it comfortably. Besides, I don't want to work that hard.

Flooding is different from a phobic reaction, though sometimes the two are confused. The overstimulation is not symbolic or "abnormal." It is a reasonable response of a sensitive person. Simply let your reactions be your guide, and you will feel a lot better.

Confusion may be your response to being blamed for things about which you have no idea what to do. Especially if you are not aware of your style of brain construction and aren't trained to deal with it in your everyday world, you become susceptible to scolding, put downs, and even physical or verbal punishment, such as being asked "Why didn't you do what I told you?" when you had no idea why.

As a result, you may experience feelings of helplessness when you don't understand what went wrong. You will likely have no idea what you could have done to change the situation. This is why training to understand your ADD and utilize your skills effectively is so important. You can learn to avoid feelings of utter hopelessness.

But until you have the skills to deal with your brainstyle, know that there is a reason for the ways you feel. Trust yourself. Quickly come to know the limitations and strengths of your brainstyle. Don't promise what you can't do or don't habitually follow through on. If you make a commitment, make it small and implement it NOW. Never say, "I'll do so and so later."

Take one small step at a time and ask the others in your life to also become knowledgeable about ADD. If you're not moving quickly enough for them, set a limit and say, "I am doing what I can do. If it is not fast enough for you, then I ask you to get some help with your needs." Invariably, I've discovered that when a person with an ADD style begins to do self-work, a partner may become very angry and unwittingly sabotage the changes being made. It's up to you to be firm in the best interest of both of you.

This is the same pattern that is seen in addiction and codependency treatment. The person who looked okay turns out to have a role in the selection of a companion who is compromised. When the "identified patient" begins to change for the better, the original reasons surface for the partner selecting someone with problems as a mate.

Anger is the first response, and denial runs rampant, too. If you're cleaning up your act, be prepared to continue your work rather than regressing to playing out the role of the incompetent one who is nagged and scolded by your partner so he or she can remain "top dog" and again appear responsible on the surface. This is tough work, and couples counseling is strongly recommended.

Impulsivity, often linked to sensitivity, is also often misperceived. True, it must be mastered so that it doesn't get you in trouble. But the first step is to understand the origins of the behavior. Then you can truly treat the cause(s) instead of simply topically attempting to treat the symptom.

Consider the case of Lenny, a 23-year-old college graduate who'd always been a bit of a hothead. However, he'd turned into a very good salesman. He liked selling and liked his job until recently, when his old boss was transferred and a new one moved in.

The old boss was a kind, compassionate man who trusted Lenny, and if he had something to say to Lenny, he never sounded like he was criticizing him. And he extended generosity to other salespeople.

Sales reports were normally due by two o'clock Friday, but the boss extended the deadline for one salesman, who always had lunch with his daughter on Friday. The salesman was divorced and missed his daughter very much, and lunching with her was important to him. Extending the report deadline for him was no problem for anyone.

When the new boss came on board, it was another story. The man was a critical, toe-the-line kind of guy who raised his voice whether he needed to or not and felt obligated to point out that he was boss. Even before he got to know anyone, he started handing out orders. Reports—all reports—had to be in by two o'clock on Friday. When the salesman who had lunch with his daughter politely asked for an extension of one hour, explaining the circumstances, the new boss gruffly replied, "No extensions, no exceptions. A job is a job, and if you can't do it, I'll find someone who can."

All the other salespeople in the office glanced at each other but stayed quiet, burying their heads in their work. But Lenny, who already felt annoyed by the sound of the man's voice and attitude, couldn't stand it. It wasn't fair to his coworker. No one else cared if the salesman's report was in by two o'clock.

Lenny got up and walked over to the new boss and right in front of everyone said, "That's not right. You shouldn't have done that. He's a good worker and it doesn't hurt anyone to extend his deadline. You have no right to do it."

The boss yelled, "Sit down!" and Lenny stalked out of the office yelling, "You're crazy. You got no right to come in here and treat people that way. We were doing fine before you came."

When a friend tried to talk to him later, he was still hot under the collar and refused to apologize or back off. In fact, he quit the next day, when upon returning to pick up his worksheet for the day, he ran into his boss, who demanded an apology and started to lecture him. Lenny exploded and walked out.

Understandable. But did he really help his friend? And what did he do to his own life and to his family?

The trick that Lenny needs to learn is to use his anger and righteousness in a way that truly can make a difference.

- First and foremost, he needs to learn to quietly back away and get out of the line of the source of his pain.

- Next, he must do nothing until he cools off.

- Once cooled off, it would do him good to get together with others in his group and begin to strategize in relation to the situation. Numerous heads are better than one.

- Once he or they have a plan that's been well thought through, they can decide how to implement it.

- If the boss is at all approachable, it behooves him or them to make an appointment to talk the situation over to see if a peaceful resolution can be reached.

- If it is not possible, then there is always the option of going above the new boss to see if anything can be done.

- If that is not possible or is nonproductive, Lenny and his colleagues must decide what they personally want to do about it. This could be the time to lay the groundwork for a transfer within the company. Or it could be time to seek a new job.

The important thing in situations like this is to keep the timing and moves under your control so that you don't reap penalties for hasty behavior. There's nothing wrong with holding tight to your beliefs and standing up on principle. But it's all in the way you do it. Impulsive actions rob you of your power and reduce the likelihood that you'll make a difference in the long run.

The Group Effect

One other treatment option I wish to mention is making use of the Group Effect. When ADD has gone unrecognized in childhood, the initial reaction in an adult is relief: relief at finding an explanation for much of what has caused disruption and unfulfilled potential in a person's life. Euphoria may accompany relief. Whew! It feels as if anything is possible.

At this point, it is good to talk with others about your awareness of ADD. The discussion will help ground you until there is time to catch up with your new identity.

Some communities will have a self-help clearinghouse and a guide to local services. Community colleges and psychologist's and physician's offices may know of resources, or the Mental Health Association may be a place to start. Of course, look on the Internet to see if you can find any local groups with which to connect. Schools may help you make contact with the parents of children with an ADD brainstyle.

Find one of these groups and consider joining. Then you can sort through the many options you have for dealing with your needs and wishes. This will provide you with choices, as a group of people will reflect the many ways that people have found to deal with ADD. If you find no group, form your own. That's what we initially did in Dallas in the early 1990s, and that's what we're again doing via the Internet over a decade later. (See appendix E for the website.)

Remember that you are seeking information to make choices for yourself. You will see that you share a common bond of experience with others. But you may also see that you are different in many ways in your response to your awareness of being ADD.

If you're creative or using your ADD to advantage, you may only be seeking tips on how to handle a small area of your life, such as accounting or linear learning situations. If you need a more structured approach, you may be able to find a training program. You can get the scoop on the pros and cons of medication; you can seek a mentor if you wish. If you are having relationship or marriage problems, you can get advice in that arena or find a group for you and your committed other or for that other person by herself or himself.

Your group will care about you. Use them to learn new ways. Learn to see yourself as you are and work to change what you don't like. But throughout this phase, be very careful to avoid thinking you are pathological or ought to change the roots of your innate self. Keep your ADD, but modify the aspects of your life that you would like to change. This gives your Accommodating Self a head start on connecting fully with your True Self. It's your choice.

Treating the abuse and inner pain that is often a part of having an ADD style of brain construction is one of the best gifts you can give yourself. Pick and choose the elements you wish to use. Think about this phase of "treatment" as a journey back to the perfect, wonderful person you were always meant to be: your True Self. And know that you can learn to utilize your special way of being to the benefit of yourself, your family, and your community.

5

TREATING ABUSE AND INNER PAIN

The very name of the ADD brainstyle perpetrates abuse and causes inner pain. By virtue of being called "deficit" or "disordered," there is a residue of feelings of inadequacy in everyone I've ever met who has a significant number of ADD attributes. Being required to be labeled as "handicapped" in order to be given equal opportunity to access educational and work opportunities is a case in point. This is true even if you've learned to use your attributes successfully. Abuse of people with ADD attributes comes in many forms:

- Being told, "You can do it if you just try," when in fact you can't.
- Being told, "You never follow through," when the focus is on linear tasks.
- Being told, "You're too sensitive," when, in fact, empathy and compassion are stellar values.

- Being forced to sit for hours to learn something, when you could learn it standing or walking around.

- Being denied the opportunity to "show your stuff" because the test to show what you know is of a nature that doesn't fit your brainstyle, regardless of whether you can do the job or not.

- Being insensitively treated, even if unwittingly. (The bed sheets may have felt abrasive to you as an infant with your sensitive skin.)

- Being continually pressured to do what doesn't fit you or reaps disapproval, disappointment, or even punishment, even when what you're being asked to do doesn't interest you.

- Being denied educational opportunities to utilize the brainpower you have, even though you could learn from the use of nonlinear (analog) learning techniques, leading to feelings of being abused.

The accumulation of hundreds of such events—subtle sometimes, harsh at other times—leads to deep, lasting pain. The expression of abuse takes both physical and emotional forms. Take the case of George, a successful salesman who starts drinking every day at noon. As a child, he'd been labeled lazy and was repeatedly punished at home and at school for not finishing his schoolwork. Without alcohol, he feels the pain of the switchings and rapped knuckles, the humiliation, and the anxiety of childhood every time he enters a place of business. George was the victim of physical and emotional abuse.

Or take Jennifer, who has been in an entry-level civil service position for five years, despite having a college degree. She has low self-esteem and doesn't believe she's capable of doing any better, so she puts out little effort. She was often told she was dumb and would never be able to do the simplest of jobs. So Jennifer does just what she is told, never tries any more than the simplest of jobs. Her abuse is the result of words.

In addition to the self-depreciation that words and poor job performance create, there are subtle actions and blatant actions that strike at the heart and soul of someone with a brainstyle that doesn't fit someone else's perception of what is the right way to be. Usually, the responsibility for fixing the problem a child has with behavior and learning is placed on the child, regardless of his or her age. The parents and teachers press the child for results in the improvement of their behavior when they, the adults, don't know what to do to make the situation better. I've never understood this. If the adults don't know what to do, how in the world is the child to know?

There's the whole realm of adult responses, from arched eyebrows to scolding, to grounding, to time out, to missed recess and extracurricular activities. In addition, there's severe guilt-producing verbiage about the lack of caring and goodness of the child and, finally, physical punishment that borders on abuse and sometimes crosses the line, becoming physical abuse. All of these responses to a child's behavior leave marks on the psyche of a child. To grow in a healthy way, these wounds must be healed.

WHAT'S TO BE DONE ABOUT THE ABUSE AND INNER PAIN?

Because of the sensitivity of people with an ADD style of brain construction (remember Sherry), it is important to tread carefully and gently on our psyches. Sledgehammers are rarely needed. Firmness, yes, but not further abuse at the hands of

Lisa's Story: Healing the Wounds Within

Lisa's dream was to be like Karla. That was in fourth grade. Thirty-two years later, she no longer tries to be like Karla.

Karla was *so* sweet. She could be quiet, she could sit still, and all her teachers loved her. She never had to try to get people to like her. Lisa, in contrast, spent her time acting up, getting into fights, or not paying attention. She was blamed for not being able to be like other kids and got in trouble for trying to be like them. She was isolated from other children much of the time as punishment.

"You're weird," people would say. Lisa was simply never able to "shut such things out." She needed to defend herself and other underdogs.

But Lisa made it through high school, and though she immediately found a place for herself working in radio, it took time until she could get beyond the voices in her head that repeatedly told her she was behind and always would be. She noticed in her late teens and early twenties that others could stay on a path and travel straight to a goal. "Me, I'd go to the right, then to the left, and then get back on the path."

She thought this was the wrong way to be, that if she could travel a straight line, she would be farther ahead than she was. Then she would mentally beat herself up. As a result, she experienced her world as too painful, so much so that "I got into a lot of *stuff* that I shouldn't have—to tone down the pain."

Ironically, it was when she got her own talk radio show and began interviewing guests about Attention Deficit Disorder that Lisa discovered why she had difficulty staying on a straight path. She recognized her *outrageous* behavior in other media people with whom she worked. Many shared the same difficulties she'd encountered over the years. In the talk show business, she found kindred spirits.

Discovering why school was so hard and why she didn't seem to fit presented her with choices. If she chose to *treat* her ADD, she feared she'd lose the edge she had in the entertainment business. She, and others, loved her spontaneity and quickness. She realized that the fact that she didn't stay on the straight path efficiently actually provided her with material for her general-interest shows. Her curiosity, allowed to run free, made for great programs. Improvisation was her forte.

So she chose to not use medication. And she embraced her ADD attributes as a gift—her talent, the very lifeblood of what she loved to do. And she gave herself permission to engage in what she loved, recognizing it was because of her ADD.

To be sure, not all has been sweetness and light for Lisa on her way up the entertainment ladder. As a young DJ, she found so much going on at the local station that there was always something to hold her attention. She was able to keep focused on the tasks. But when she was promoted, she had technical assistants to do many of the tasks she'd previously done. It was then that she ran into trouble. She had less to do that held her attention, so she found herself drifting off during the songs, since they were all she had to concentrate on.

When she got her own talk show, her attention was easily held during the show—it was a job designed for people who multitask. She loved being on the air, but preparing for the show was something else. She'd get distracted at home going through all the latest local and national newspapers because she couldn't concentrate on one story at a time. Her creative mind jumped to attention with each new bit of information, ever creating new programming ideas.

Discovering that she had an ADD style of brain construction, Lisa found ways to work with her attention in user-unfriendly situations. She read a lot about ADD and created her own tips to help her maneuver through non-ADD minefields. When she failed or found something inordinately difficult or not to her taste, she asked for help, instead of beating up on herself.

Harder to deal with, however, were her bad feelings from childhood. As with all victims of abuse, Lisa blamed herself. She knew that ignoring the pain or trying to cover it with substances didn't work. Instead, conjuring an image of the scenes from her past, she befriended the little memory-child who envied Karla. She firmly stood up for herself. She imagined giving information about brain construction to Karla, her teachers, and others who had blamed her for the way she was constructed. She designed a new, more appropriate learning environment for her school-age self. She saw the teachers, kids, and her parents change toward her. She was then able to forgive them and envision a new outcome—the kind that follows understanding where everyone is valued.

The result of Lisa's healing work was release from feelings of pain and inadequacy. Being called "outrageous" became a compliment. After treatment, Lisa began to give herself permission to be who she was and to feel valuable as a result.

Lisa made choices that used her ADD in a positive manner and let her natural self blossom. It took understanding about her unique style of brain construction to begin the process of self-forgiveness. She consciously forgave herself and those who had failed to understand her during earlier years. Now, rather than concentrating on what she can't or hadn't been able to do, Lisa focuses on what she can do.

She has learned to treasure herself and wouldn't want to be any other way than the way she is. After all, it's her ADD attributes that provide her with professional and personal success so she can live the way she wants to and no longer has to worry.

therapists, counselors, and other well-wishers who don't understand us. This includes intense behavior modification to "get" you to act in a linear fashion.

Traditional psychotherapy often does not work well for the treatment of ADD. If you are sensitive, you may need to buffer yourself from too much insight or too many feelings being stirred up all at once. You don't need painful feelings ground into your already hurt emotional system. You already know what emotions feel like. For that reason, cognitive thinking therapy that gives you information may work better than feelings-oriented therapy.

THE VISUALIZATION TECHNIQUE

There are those of you reading this book whose pain is indeed great from your growing-up years. Hurt, abuse, and anger—and more hurt—were so monumental you couldn't escape them, let alone do anything about them. Remember, abuse from ADD may have resulted from benign circumstances, but nonetheless it was there. A legacy may remain from teachers, parents, and employers whose personal goals—to train you properly—were thwarted by your having an ADD style of brain construction.

The abuse may have come in the form of well-meant scoldings or behavioral limits that you couldn't abide, such as groundings or being kept after school. Of course, at times, the abuse may have been much more than that, including overreactive responses such as physical punishment and beatings.

For you, I want to suggest that you practice a technique used in many fields, for many purposes: visualization. I have made modifications to the technique that I originally used treating post-traumatic stress disorder, to make that technique more appropriate and successful for ADD treatment. Look at it as a tool for "reparenting" yourself or, if you prefer, "re-experiencing" your past.

In a quiet place, sit in a comfortable chair that has arms, close your eyes, and take a step back from your experience. Think of something that makes you feel secure, safe, and protected. It might be sitting in the lap of your grandmother. Or it might be feeling the sun on your shoulders while you walk through a forest filled with the smell of springtime, with a soft breeze playing against your cheek. Choose your own brand of safety—and feel the arm of the chair.

Imagine projecting your experience onto a movie screen, and view it as you might a movie. As you do this, grasp the arm of the chair that you're sitting in while watching the movie, and feel the security of it. You can even see yourself watching the movie.

(*If you feel resistant to doing this exercise, don't do it. Your psyche is telling you: "Whoa, this is not good for me." You may wish to do this work with a counselor or not at all. Your psyche knows best. Trust it.*)

Let your mind drift back to a time in your youth when you felt misunderstood, inadequate, or out of control. Visualize that part of you in your mind's eye. You will probably feel a sensation within you that reflects how you felt at the time. Pay particular attention to that feeling, its shape, its location in your physical body, and its size and substance. Is it hot or cold, hard or soft, solid or porous? Attach a color to it.

Immediately after defining this feeling, squeeze the arm of the chair and find that nice, warm secure feeling. As you neutralize the sensation that causes you discomfort, realize that you can grow beyond your history.

Remember, if you are projecting this experience on a movie screen, keep it there while you watch yourself sitting and watching the movie.

Next, let your mind drift back to an earlier time in your life when you encountered a similar feeling. Locate its presence in your body again, and visualize where you were standing as a child when it happened. What were you doing? Squeeze the arm of the chair. Remember to keep the vision on your movie screen.

Now, go back and seek the earliest experience you can recall when the same constellation of events or feelings took place. You may have been four, five, or six years old. Once more, squeeze the arm of the chair and check your movie screen if you need to.

It is now time to rewrite your history.

Pretend you are a scriptwriter. You have the capability to rewrite your childhood history any way you want. You can give your child words and understanding that he or she would not have had. In this rewriting job, anything is possible. Also allow the others in your drama to have words, skills, and understanding they didn't actually have but that you can give them since you are recreating their characters.

Visualize your child self with the out-of-control, inadequate feelings and let the child say what he or she needs: Understanding from others? Support of others? A sense of control in the situation? Your child self might say something like: "I feel overwhelmed. I need you to understand that I'm trying as hard as I can." Squeeze the arm of the chair you're sitting in. Feel it holding you up.

Visualize the grown-ups in your life reassuring you as a child, giving you understanding, knowledge, or whatever you needed. Hear them teaching your child self: "You have an ADD brain. That's great. Sometimes it creates a problem, though. I can help you learn to overcome any problems that do come up. You are smart. You are okay. I love you. I'm here with you, and I'll help you learn in your special way. See, you are already doing it. You're a fast learner. I love you."

If you like, feel the warm arm of the adult around your child shoulders. Watch the adult walk you into school and explain to the teachers what is needed. See the teachers pass the message on. And see your child grow assured, secure, capable, and able to be in control.

If the adults in your early life were particularly abusive, see your child self on the movie screen stop them. Have them freeze like the child's game, "freeze," where no one can move without permission of the game leader. Let your child self be the leader and call "freeze." Then let a special, understanding adult teach them about ADD.

Next, watch the abusive adults change their level of understanding as they are enlightened. Let them say, "I am so sorry. I didn't mean you any harm. I didn't know any better. Please forgive me."

Watch the child on the screen take as long as he needs to forgive. No rush. If your child self needs to vent some anger, fine. If the child wants to scold, fine. When the feeling is vented and you see the adults for what they were—frightened, helpless, frustrated—forgiveness will come. But let it come in its own time as you again squeeze the arm of your chair, feeling the security it offers, as well as the support and comfort.

Feel the child's growing sense of control. Realize that the feeling will spread and grow to be used daily as you go about your business in confidence, knowing that you are now understood and strong.

You can change each recalled experience this way. Give your child within what is needed. Provide the child with the power of information and the support of understanding. Watch the child, adolescent, and adult in you grow in confidence before your mind's eye. Forgive those who hurt you out of ignorance and feel confidence build within you so you can be in control of yourself as someone who is ADD.

COMMON QUESTIONS ABOUT VISUALIZATION

What can I do if I can't get my mind to be quiet enough to do the visualization?

- Make sure that you get into a regular daily habit of spending time quietly so that your mind and emotions can count on the time.
- Make a list of intruding concerns and problems that are most likely to distract you and commit to return to them at a later time.
- Slow your breathing down and feel it becoming a little deeper and more regular.
- Experiment to see which is easiest for you, closing your eyes, keeping your eyes open, or keeping your eyes open but focusing on one thing.
- Clear your mind further by letting a gentle breeze carry your thoughts off, by taking a mental broom and sweeping

them aside, or by placing them on a shelf or in a box for later sorting.

Start the visualization but don't expect to finish it. Do it in stages, being easy on yourself.

What should I do if I start feeling very emotional during the visualization?

Stop. Don't go further into it.

Allow yourself to stay with the feeling. Be gentle and nurturing with yourself. Express the feeling out loud to yourself, letting the adult part of you realize that your little kid part was deeply touched.

You may not want to do any further work with the visualization that day. You may want to talk with someone about the feelings. Do so. Return to the visualization at a time when it feels comfortable to do so.

What do I do if I have trouble seeing pictures in my mind or don't see them at all? Does that mean there is something else wrong with me?

There is nothing wrong with you. Some people visualize easily. Other people are better at hearing dialogue in their heads. And still others do best feeling things.

If you are having trouble getting pictures in your mind, try having a conversation with yourself and your inner child. Recall the conversations you had as a child, and remember what you heard that impressed you.

If this method still leaves you wanting, settle on feeling the experiences that you went through as a child and substitute the feelings you would have liked that child to have had. Bring the child feelings of joy and power. You can do this by recalling feelings of joy and power in other settings and transferring those feelings to your ADD experience.

When the history of my childhood is being rewritten, what do I do if I simply can't see my parents being helpful?

Some people have to substitute other people for their parents. It may be an aunt or uncle, family friend, doctor, public figure, or someone from literature. Call forth the person you would have liked to have had as a parent. Some people who are parents themselves visualize their adult selves taking care of their child selves, saying, "I wish I'd had a parent like me."

When I do the visualization and let myself experience the child, I get angry—very, very angry. How do I handle that?

If you feel your anger could get out of control, protect yourself and others by doing the visualization with someone else present. A counselor can help you with this.

Often, however, we feel that any anger at all is a lot. This happens if we were raised with a prohibition on the expression of any anger, or if we viewed a family member getting out of control with his or her anger. In that case, you might try feeling a little bit of it by yourself. But be kind to yourself, and call on a friend if you're concerned.

There is nothing wrong with screaming, shouting, or stomping your anger out on the ground. It's only a feeling. It's only anger. Try kicking a stone down the street, playing racquetball or handball, throwing a pillow, or saying some four-letter words.

Do I need to confront the people in real life who hurt me?

No. Usually the hurt was done out of ignorance. You will be farther ahead in your healing process if you acknowledge the hurts and errors and absorb yourself in fixing them.

If your abusers are open to learning, share the information you have with them. Do this is in a matter-of-fact way. You will know if you feel strongly about confronting them. Do so if you wish, but only after you've focused on what you can do and paid attention to what shaped that person's behavior. You may wish to say something such as, "I understand that you were abused as a child. I realize that when you hurt me, you hadn't taken responsibility for your healing, and you took your hurt out on me. I also want you to know what you did was wrong. I didn't deserve it, and I feel angry (if you do) about what you did. I would like an apology (if, in fact, you do want one)."

Then decide what you want to do next. You may want to walk away and not be involved with that person again. Or you may want to explore further healing between you. You will know what you want and are ready to do.

Remember, the main job is to heal yourself and take over responsibility for your growth.

Why is it so hard to forgive and go on?

All of us have a hard time living with unfinished emotional business. Our emotions keep pulling us back to the problem in an attempt to get us to solve it. Usually, we don't let go of a problem because there is some aspect that is not yet solved. People with ADD have to work hard to get past the point of hurt or blame and turn that energy into constructive action. But it is worth the effort.

How long will it take for my inner child to forgive those who abused me?

It will take your child part as long as it needs to take. There is no point in pushing yourself. Do not let others try to tell you that you *should* forgive your abusers. It will simply happen when all the healing is done.

What if I can't get my inner child to forgive them?

Often, unexpressed anger stands in the way of being able to forgive someone. This is most likely to happen when we understand what happened to us but have not yet fully felt or acknowledged all the feelings within. It's a matter of getting what we know cognitively to the level of feelings. Once the feelings are fully acknowledged and felt, and appropriate action is taken on behalf of them, the forgiveness comes automatically.

How long will it take me to go through the grief process about having been abused and hurt?

Grieving also takes as long as it takes. A major grief reaction (following divorce or the death of a loved one) takes at least two years. Recovery from grief over your lost potential may go more quickly, provided you work with it. One reason is that you haven't been permanently separated from your potential. Rather you have been blocked from accessing it, but it has been waiting for you to make it safe enough for it to resurface. Doing the visualization work will facilitate your recovery, and it may take only a session or two to get beyond the feelings you've carried all these years. Don't worry, though, if it takes longer.

What does it mean if I don't or can't feel any grief over my lost potential?

You may have already gone through your grief. You certainly don't want to make up feelings you don't have.

How can I learn to let myself feel?

Begin with another person who will help you realize *when* you are feeling. That person can be a counselor but doesn't necessarily have to be. She can be a friend who will stop you when you get an expression on your face or act in a way that tells her you are having feelings. You can then learn to identify what you were feeling.

If I start letting myself feel, will I still be able to work and stay in control of my life?

Of course. In fact, you will be even more in control, because it is an illusion that your feelings will go away if you don't acknowledge them. They actually only get more out of control, doing their work behind the scenes.

To protect other areas of your life from the effects of your feelings, you can assign specific times to pay attention to them separate from work. Compartmentalize. Let your inner child know you will come back to the feelings at the specific time you've set aside to deal with them.

I'm shy around other people and wouldn't want to let other people know what I really feel. Can I fix myself in private?

You can begin to work with your feelings in private, but ultimately you will benefit from openly acknowledging them.

Being reticent with your feelings is one of the symptoms of the hurt and emotional damage you have suffered.

Shame is one of the most common reactions to such hurt, leaving us feeling as if others would reject us or not want to be around us if they really knew what we felt or were like. Not so!

You were not responsible for what happened to you. Let awareness of this rescue you from feelings of self-blame. Be as firm with yourself as you are with anyone else who tries to make you responsible for being made the way you are. You are, and have always been, just fine as you are.

If I don't feel comfortable doing the visualization, how can I feel better about myself?

There are many ways to heal the past so you can move on to the future. You may be able to write out your healing. Try writing a letter to the child within you who suffered the repercussions of ADD. Also write letters to those who hurt you and to those who helped you. You can get your anger out this way and can even write a letter forgiving everyone involved, but only when you are good and ready. You may or may not send these letters. The writing of them may be enough. Decide what to do with them based on what you feel you want to do, not on what you think you *should* do.

I've known people who painted out their healing and others who used athletics, music, drama, and gardening. Anything goes. Use the mode that you feel drawn to.

How can I like the child part of me? She's so dumb.

You have a good case of self-abuse going. Realize you learned to feel that way, so you can unlearn it. Try getting a picture of yourself when you were about five or six. That's probably when you started school and began to have trouble with your ADD. Talk with the child in the picture.

Share the picture with someone you trust. Often a therapist can help you with this phase, especially if you have a tough case of "dumb feelings." As the other person loves your child, you will have a model to watch and imitate. The day will come, mark my words, when you will appreciate your child and understand her pain. You will then look at her as a courageous person who survived.

I can't get over feeling bad about having trouble in school and everyone blaming me.

The most common block in this kind of situation is unexpressed anger. In your mind, call forth the people who offended you and let the schoolchild tell them off royally.

See your child being taught in a way that fits her brainstyle. Then visualize the child going through school successfully, with understanding from the adults and other children. In fact, have them congratulate her on her assets while she helps them with their deficits.

6

TRAINING: AN ALTERNATIVE WAY OUT

The question raised in the previous chapter, "What shall I do about how I am constructed?" suggested two options: treatment and training. Training does not attempt to alter your innate brainstyle, but tries instead to make it work more effectively for you. Then you can go after any goal that is generally thought to be important, and you can do it in any way that uses your strengths.

In this chapter, we'll look at some of the training options that are available to you. They are based on three themes that describe the situations faced by anyone with a diverse brain construction. These are: the True You, the Wounded You, and the Accommodating You. The Wounded You was covered earlier in this book, in the introduction.

The True You is the style of brain construction with which you were born. It is the natural style that brings with it assets and liabilities as any style does. What lay previously undetected or underdeveloped can be embraced and used in your personal and work life for the benefit of all. The True You is the unwarped, unjudged, unwounded, natural you.

I ask you to focus on the way in which you think, act, and express yourself. You can reach any goals of importance to you in ways that fit your natural bent. All you need to do is notice your feelings of enthusiasm or hesitation when tackling an activity or situation. You will be drawn to activities and situations that are right for you, that support your natural skills, and that provide you with a sense that you can reach your potential. You'll learn to recognize your hesitation to engage in activities and situations that don't naturally fit you and that are not good for you. From this approach, you'll come to know meaningful success.

As you become aware of the True You, you will learn to recognize how well your surroundings fit you. You'll become attuned to beliefs that honor you. While you are searching for the true environment of the True You, you will need to continue to respond the best you can to situations that are not a good match for how you are made. You will do this until you can do what is needed to make a better fit possible. This takes time.

The Accommodating You will make contact with the imperfect world we encounter in everyday life. Living in an imperfect world means you will not always be able to find a fit between your natural ways and the environments you face. But you can learn skills to bridge the differences between your innate skills and the expectations placed on you. And you can do that without hurting yourself further.

You, too, can achieve through training whether you have a few or many ADD attributes. You can learn to make maximum use of your True Self. And you can find ways your Accommodating Self can function using natural ADD skills to achieve linear results. For example, if you are trying to organize something—something that is not easy for most ADD folks to do—it's probably because you've been taught only linear ways to do the job. You, too, can become organized when you learn to sort, file, and handle projects in an ADD, nonlinear way. That's what *The New Attention Deficit Disorder in Adults Workbook* helps you to do. For now, I'll include a few samples to get you started. I expect that you'll be convinced to keep on building your reservoir of skills so you can truly achieve in a manner that is comfortable for you.

Ready? Let's look at training options that will reinforce and make use of your innate characteristics and that will help you to accommodate situations that are not a natural fit.

- You have either come to the conclusion that you have a number of ADD attributes through self-assessment, or you have been formally assessed by a professional and given the label of Attention Deficit Disorder.
- Next decide how you want to approach the handling of your new awareness.
- Finally, look at your training options. Decide which option you wish to begin with.
    - Workbook-guided training
    - Group training

Let your feelings and needs guide you in making a choice about which of these to pursue at first. You can do both or start one and switch to the other. You're in charge.

Titus's Story: ADD: Hope for a New Life

A young man in prison khakis walks toward me down a dimly lit hall. We're in the education building of a low-security prison.

Even before I can clearly see his features, I notice his swagger. Every part of his body moves as he walks. His head tosses errant hair back from his forehead, his arms churn, his hips sway, and his gait proclaims loudly that he is on a mission.

"Hmmmm," I think, assessing what I see. His silent bravado proclaims his inner sensitivity and insecurity about our scheduled meeting. None of this is new to me in this setting. "Is she to be trusted?" is the critical first thought in any first-time meeting that takes place in prison.

I reach out my hand and say, "Hi. You're Titus, aren't you? I'm Lynn Weiss." The twenty-year-old takes my hand almost reluctantly, but quickly responds to my firm, sure grip. It is as if in the flash of an eye, he sees something he can trust in me—maybe just a little.

His GED teacher has referred him to me because he was "driving her nuts." Seems he moves his chair close to the wall and tilts it backward so he can rock back and forth while he attempts to do his studies. When she tells him to put all four legs of the chair on the floor, he does it . . . for about five seconds, and then the next thing she knows he's tilting backward and rocking again.

He is teetering on the edge of getting himself thrown into the "hole." That means he is in danger of being locked up 24 hours a day in a tiny cell that will cause him to miss school and work from which he earns money. He'll also lose "good time," which will delay his release.

In 1998, I introduced an ADD skill-building group for inmates into the prison. The teacher was very aware of ADD characteristics and had decided to refer Titus both to the group and for individual work with me before writing him up.

"He's not a bad guy," she told me. "Some are. He's not. He's young and not mean, but he's sure not learning. In fact, his GED pretest scores are plummeting instead of improving." Then, in an offhand comment, she added, "You know, he seems to do better work when he's rocking."

It made sense immediately.

With this in mind, I smile at Titus and ask, "What's the deal with your chair-rocking business?" Then, I add, "You know it's making your teacher nuts, and that's not good for her or you." With that, I look him directly in the eye with a little twinkle showing in mine.

He flashes a smile, then a frown, and begins with a drawl, "Well . . ." He hesitates.

I jump in and say, "Titus, look, whatever you say is confidential. I think you're a good guy, but there's some reason you keep doing what your teacher doesn't want, and it's my job to figure out the reason. It will be your job to use what I find out so you can stop messing up and stay out of trouble. Okay? Got it?"

Titus nods, and his bright eyes look straight at me. He understands.

"I'm not trying to hassle my teacher. Mostly I don't even know I'm doing it."

"Mostly?" I query.

He grins. "Sometimes I do it on purpose when I'm bored."

I respond half seriously and half jokingly, "Whew, that's a high price for reducing boredom—if you keep it up and lose good time! But," I shrug, "that's your choice." My voice is nonjudgmental as I state a reality of prison life.

At that, Titus gets serious and says, "I don't want to get into trouble here. But I kinda feel it's hopeless. I'm trying hard, but no matter how much I want to do good, I do something like tip my chair back when I don't even mean to do it. My pretest scores are even going down."

Over the next few weeks, Titus and I meet weekly, and he also attends an ADD skill-building group that teaches him how brain construction affects his behavior, his interests, and his ability to do his schoolwork. He learns many of the techniques included in this book. He proves to be an avid worker and quick learner. As a result, he begins to be in control and achieve success.

Almost immediately, he stops tilting his chair. Because he learns better when he's active, we focus on his learning to use alternative ways to move around while he is in class. He learns to break his assignments into manageable pieces. He discovers ways to keep his attention on his schoolwork. His pretest scores begin to rise.

Titus's swagger disappears, and he becomes less volatile when touched or surprised. He not only comes to understand about his sensitivity, but he also practices ways to get what he needs while both protecting himself and staying out of trouble.

Three months later, his teacher reports, with a catch in her voice, that Titus has passed the GED exam. Word comes from the guards that he no longer causes trouble in the unit, mess hall, and rec yard. He is promoted to a better-paying job in prison industries. He begins to save the money he earns for when he is released. He's considering taking college-level correspondence courses. He's even beginning to think about what he might like to do when he is released from prison. Perhaps he will end up teaching others what he has learned. Time will tell. Titus has hope.

WORKBOOK-GUIDED TRAINING: TRAIN YOURSELF

If you opt for workbook-guided training, I refer you to *The New Attention Deficit Disorder in Adults Workbook*. You can work with this book by yourself or with a partner. Of course, you can also use it in a group setting. Work at your own speed and use as much of it as you wish.

Here are several examples of typical issues with which people with an ADD brainstyle appreciate getting help.

Skill 1: Procrastination

Procrastination is an organizational issue, and a characteristic that is generally looked at negatively. And it certainly has its downside when deadlines are missed. But there is another way to look at procrastination.

Background: The step-by-step linear way of proceeding does not fit an ADD brainstyle. Generally, as an ADD person, you will not want to do an outline, at least not until your task is completed. Then, whether there is an outline or not, you will not be likely to start the task on the first day, and for sure, you won't do an equal amount on each day until the task is due. That's not a natural ADD way.

Why this happens: If you've a lot of ADD characteristics, you are a *big-picture* person who has to see the *whole picture* of whatever you're doing before you can break out the details. Only when we see the way the elements of the pattern are put together can we describe them in outline form. You also will not start right after you've been assigned the task, even when you are the one deciding to do it. You've internal mental work to do. Sometimes this internal work is unknown to your conscious mind. But it is going on anyway. And you will start writing when it *feels* right.

Know you tend to learn kinesthetically, which means by doing a task. It usually takes a few times to get it right, but once you've learned the pattern by having done it, you've got it forever.

What to do: Write in "Yes" or "No" or other appropriate answers to the following questions and follow all steps.

1. Are you sure you are willing to do the project? _____

2. Do you give yourself permission to work on the project in your own way in your own time? _____

3. Do you understand the parameters of the assignment?___

   ____

   Who are you doing the project for? __________________

   ____

   What do you need to get across in it? ________________

   ____

   ____

   How long does it need to be? ______________________

   How long do you estimate it will take you to do it if you do it all at once? ______________________________

   Why do you think this? ___________________________

   ____

4. Do you like to work for a while, take a break, then work for a while again? ______

5. Look at a month-at-a-glance calendar and mark when the project is due. Mark in breaks you wish to take.

6. How long can you work at a sitting? _________________

7. How many days can you work without taking a break? ____________

8. How long do you want to spend working on the actual construction of this project? ____________

9. Now you'll know when you probably need to begin the actual production.

10. Throw in a few extra hours or days for good measure.

11. Do you like to work without breaks? ______

12. Don't try to equally break down the time you're committing to the project. Average your time.

13. Will you please check this estimate with your feelings later? ______

14. Are there any special preparations you need to make, special materials to order, people to interview, or research to undertake?

    Note them. ____
    ____
    ____

15. Mark your calendar when you want to do them, not when you think you ought to.

16. Now put the project in the back of your mind.

17. Do your tasks at the assigned times, but don't push the writing or production until you feel it's time to start.

18. When the time comes to begin work, review your parameters. Who, what, how? ______________________________
    ____

19. Take a deep breath, close your eyes, and ask your creative self to begin the process.

20. What picture, word, or thought jumps into your mind?
____
____

21. You're off and running. You've started.

22. Does the whole project pretty much come out all at once, requiring little cutting and pasting? ________________

23. When you're criticized for your style, simply tell people you have the situation well in hand.

24. Use this process several times to gain efficiency and trust in it.

What's hard about this: Changing a belief about yourself and the way in which you are to work is hard. You'll have to convince yourself that it's okay to do assignments in your own way.

Skill 2: Anchoring a Drifting Mind

Anchoring is a way to help you with follow-through and stay on track.

Background: Maybe you're reading, and the next thing you know, you're at the bottom of the page but you don't know what you read. Or say you're giving a talk, get off track to tell a story, and can't recall your original train of thought.

Why this happens: As a person whose brain focuses on the interconnections and relationships between things more than on specific bits of information, you are likely to drift away from one thought to a complex of thoughts. You automatically connect what you hear with what you already know and start to *think* about it.

You may begin to think about what you're reading or speaking about in relation to yourself. Next, look to see if you're drawn off track to begin to think about yourself. You may begin to have feelings that pull you off track or bodily needs that distract you. You may get a new idea you've never had before. You may become bored, already knowing what the writer is going to say.

What to do: Don't beat up on yourself. Write "Yes" or "No" or other appropriate answers to the following questions.

1. Are you willing to learn to anchor your attention so you won't *stay* "off track" for long? ______

2. Are you willing to develop the skill of noticing when your mind drifts? ______

   If you've answered "yes" to both, continue.

3. When you are reading and your mind drifts, will you place your finger on the place in the book where you begin to think about something other than what you are reading?

   ______

4. Will you jot down a word or two or draw a picture in the column of your book to remind you of the intervening thought? ______

   Draw a picture right now of something you might be thinking about. Make it a very simple sketch. You don't have to be an artist.

5. Will you commit to return to your note or picture later?

   ______

What makes this hard to do: It takes practice to get through to your attention span to learn new habits. You must tell yourself you can do it. And you must practice for a while. Even then, you may occasionally drift. Be grateful that you're integrating new information so quickly.

Skill 3: Finding Ways to Sit Still

Jiggling your foot, tapping your fingers, and clicking your tongue are all typical ADD attributes.

Background: When you don't have an active role in what is going on, you are likely to have lots of trouble being still. You are usually effective and happy when you are moving and doing. It's one of your best characteristics. The counterside is that being still feels awful.

Some people are more expressive when they're tapping, thumping, and fidgeting. This can be quite bothersome to other people. Others are quieter and call less attention to their restlessness, but still feel bad when required to be still. It can be quite painful. In our culture, stillness is preferred to activity in many situations. Yet, as kinesthetic people, we do better when we're active.

What to do: Write "Yes" or "No" or other appropriate answers to the following questions.

1. Do you agree to learn ways to accommodate your activity level so you are comfortable and don't bother others? ______

2. Do you agree to acknowledge and accept your need for movement and be prepared ahead of time to avert problems?______

3. List things you like to do but find you have trouble being still while doing. ____

____

____

4. Think of places where you can move as you like. For example, choose a theater that has soft, big, comfortable seats. Better yet, one that has rocking seats. Where would you go? ____

____

____

5. In a meeting, will you wiggle your toes in your shoes? ____________

   Will you hide your feet under a table? ________________

   Will you cut a deal with a friend to discreetly remind you to settle down? ____________________________

   What *will* you do? ____

   ____

   ____

6. Will you agree to walk around at the back of a room if you can't sit comfortably any longer? ______

7. Visualize doing this and commit to do it the next time you are in a meeting.

8. What can you take with you that you can "fiddle with" to release pent up tension? ____________________________

____

____

____

9. How long are you able to sit before you get restless?
____

10. How can you "escape" from your work desk? _________
____
____

What makes this hard to do: Believing that any motion is wrong. Small, unobtrusive motions that relieve stress and do not bother those around you are the answer.

Skill 4: Defending the Underdog

This means you play a rescue role and often do it loudly or empathetically.

Background: Because of your sensitivity and empathy for others, you are likely to jump in to try to relieve a problem. Perhaps you rescue stray animals or cry over dead butterflies. Maybe you even fight someone you think is taking advantage of a weaker person. All this is because you feel everything so much and put yourself in the other person's shoes. It just plain hurts too much to do nothing.

What to do: Do not stop feeling or become dulled to the hurtful things in the world. Do not, however, let yourself drown in another person's problems. Write "Yes" or "No" or other appropriate answers to the following questions.

1. Are you willing to let a little time pass before you act upon your feelings? ______

2. What do you feel when you become a defender? ____
____
____

3. What situations do you feel are wrong? And how do you feel about them? Be specific. ______________________

____

____

____

4. What would be an efficient way to act? Be specific. ______

____

____

5. What can you do for someone you want to help who also won't hurt you? A win-win outcome. Be specific. _______

____

____

6. What do you want to do for someone that they can actually do for themselves? (Remember, you don't want to do anything for someone if they don't need it.) Be specific.

____

____

7. What else can you do for someone besides running in to save them? (Write an article on their behalf, refer them for help, or create an organization from which they'll benefit, etc.) Be specific. ____________________________

____

____

8. Do you need to limit your exposure to problems, such as reducing the amount of TV you watch? ______

What makes this hard to do: It's very hard for sensitive, kinesthetic people to ignore hurt and injustice. It's hard to face the fact that each of us has limitations with regard to how much we can accomplish in a lifetime to make things right. Know what you can reasonably do. Do it. Then let go of the rest.

GROUP TRAINING

If you prefer a group setting with a prescribed curriculum and a leader, then you have several choices.

Curriculum 1: Four-Week Small-Group Training

Curriculum 2: Eight- to Sixteen-Week ADD Skill-Building Program (Weiss)

Four-Week Small-Group Training Curriculum

In the education and training of adults with lots of ADD characteristics, I have discovered a short group series often works well initially. The group needs to run for a limited time to hold the interest of the participants. This kind of group can be led by anyone who has a solid, practical working knowledge of ADD in adults and good group facilitation skills. It is not necessary for the person to be a mental health professional. In fact, it often works better to have someone who's been in the trenches and has hands-on experience in running groups.

Group size: Six to eight people (it's important to not allow the group to get too big for people with ADD attributes, because a lot of interaction tends to happen).

Time: Four weeks for adults and eight weeks for adolescents.

Length of meetings: Two to three hours. The shorter groups work well in the private sector, while longer groups are needed for those who have fewer life and living skills or who must deal with chemical dependency or incarceration issues.

Format: Get-acquainted time followed by presentation of information and group discussion, personal examples, question and answer time, and special needs.

Week 1: Add 15 to 30 minutes for registration, refreshments, and get-acquainted time. Topics include:

- What it's like to be ADD. A presentation by a peer leader is especially effective here.

- Input by participants as they air their concerns about having discovered they have many ADD attributes. Personal stories are much in order here.

- Participants list special problems that they are facing on paper so leaders can be sure to incorporate problem solving into future meetings.

- A brief discussion of treatment and medication usage. A discussion of more extensive training options for skill building. You could bring someone in to talk about this if you wish.

Week 2: Handling feelings

- Present and past feelings are elicited from the participants.

- Grief work is essential in helping people with ADD characteristics grieve for the losses incurred because of ADD.

- Impulse- and temper-control techniques are taught.

- A stress-reduction/relaxation technique is taught.

Week 3: Organizational management skills

- Each participant brings examples of time-management problems from home and work. Schedules are worked up and scheduling structures are developed as date books and charts. It is important that facilitators utilize ADD-friendly ways of organizing.

- Ways to break up time are shared so that the person feels more "in control."

- Permission is given for each participant to do whatever is necessary time-wise in order to be successful. This includes leaving things to the last moment, working with the TV on, and so forth.

- Spatial management changes are developed, including the use of work carrels and other ways to break up space for more effective concentration.

- Brainstorming is used to assist individuals to come up with solutions to complicated situations. A letter may be developed for an ADD person to take to his or her boss or manager requesting special work arrangements. (The prospect of a boost in productivity is quite appealing to many employers, particularly if it is only a matter of a fairly minor adjustment that makes the difference.)

Week 4: Interpersonal relations

- Participants share specific problems with which they are confronted in their relationships at home, at school, and at work.

Communications training is presented and practiced to help ADD people get their needs met and, in turn, to meet the needs of those with whom they interact.

- Managing the "Uh-huh" phenomenon is taught; this is a commonly misunderstood response by ADD people to requests to do something, a response that lacks follow-through.

- Negotiation skills are outlined and practiced.

- The final week ends with an appraisal of the question, "Who am I if I am in charge of my life and living effectively with my wonderful ADD brainstyle?"

ADD Skill-Building Program

This program was piloted and refined at FCI–Bastrop (a minimum security federal correctional facility) in 2000. I ran similar groups throughout the '90s in varied settings: in community colleges, at ADD conferences, in private practice with clients identified with ADD attributes, and with drug- and alcohol-addicted individuals who were entered into a treatment program and given the option to simultaneously attend this skill-building group rather than be incarcerated.

It has been my experience that the background of the participants and the reason for their being in the group makes little difference in the actual curriculum material. Millionaires with impeccable records and down-and-out addicts in recovery both seem to respond positively to the material. Of course, no active drug or alcohol user is appropriate for the group, and should someone in recovery slip during the training group, they would have to immediately return to their treatment regimen or cease participating in the group.

Group size: Six to eight people (it's important to not allow the group to get too big when people with ADD attributes are involved, because a lot of interaction tends to happen).

Time: Six to twelve weeks, depending upon the interest of the participants and their additional needs, such as integrating their brainstyle material with their other issues (drugs, alcohol, crimes of impulsivity, etc.).

Length of group: Two hours.

Format: After a prescreening that coaxes out participant's ADD attributes and the specific forms of ADD, an introductory meeting is suggested that allows the participants to review the curriculum and get to know the facilitators and one another.

Week 1:

Key Attributes of ADD

Characteristics of ADD (Three Forms of ADD)

Typical Losses Due to ADD

Grief Work

Week 2:

Continuum of ADD

Traveling to a Goal

The Big Picture

Successful Goal Achievement

Week 3:

Time Usage

Time Management

R & R

The "On-Off" Switch

Week 4:

Sensitivity

Flooding

Relationships (authorities and peers)

The "Uh-huh" Phenomenon

Week 5:

The "Shoulds"

Activity Management: Physical, Verbal, Mental, Multitasking

Changing Nonconstructive Behavior: Temper Control, Impulse Control

Week 6:

What You Need to Succeed

Career Options

The Americans with Disabilities Act

29 Positive Characteristics of ADD

Celebration

The length of this group varies depending upon the interest of the participants and how deeply they wish to explore and practice their skills. One way I've found to deepen the experience is to present the material from week 1, then suggest they observe and practice the material during the week and return for a second week to go over their experiences and talk in greater depth about them.

Additional Samples of ADD Training Exercises. These exercises were taken from various ADD skill-building programs. Here are five of my all-time favorites.

- The Three-Stack Sorting Plan

  Goal: To sort through things.

  Recommend using a partner to pick up items one at a time. This reduces stress on the owner of the pile, since it eliminates choosing an item.

  Place the item in one of three stacks.

Pile 1	Pile 2	Pile 3
"I can't live without it"	*"Throw it away"*	*"I don't have a clue"*

  It may be useful to use garbage bags to pack items in each pile.

  Pile 1 must be filed, stored, moved to a new location.

Pile 2 is thrown away.

Pile 3 may be brought to a group for decision making or set aside for six months, at which time it can be assessed again using the above three categories.

- Scheduling

  Goal: To find a scheduling method that works for you.

  Try each of the following three styles of keeping track of your commitments.

- The "On-Off" Switch

  Many people with lots of ADD attributes seem to have difficulty getting started on a project. But once started, they often have an equally difficult time stopping what they are doing. It is as if the phonograph needle gets stuck in one groove and can't make it over into the next.

  Goal: To gain some control over the "On-Off" Switch.

  Steps to Working with the "On-Off" Switch:

  Step 1: Acknowledge to yourself that you often get stuck starting and stopping activities.

  Step 2: Commit to yourself to change. Say, "I want to change my behavior. I can change my behavior and become more flexible starting and stopping what I do."

  Write it. ______________________________________

  ____

  ____

DAILY ACTIVITY SCHEDULE

NAME: Jane Sample DATE: ____________________

DESCRIPTION: full time student (straight A record) who works 8 hrs per week.

	MONDAY	TUESDAY	WEDNESDAY	THURSDAY	FRIDAY	SATURDAY	SUNDAY
7:00 am	Pack Lunch Eat, Watch TV	Pack Lunch, Eat	Pack Lunch Eat, watch TV	Pack Lunch Eat	Pack Lunch Eat, watch TV	TV or sleep in work	Eat Lightly Read Book
8:00 am	↓ Drive time	Drive to school Study at	↓ Drive time	Drive to school Study at	↓ Drive Time	↓	Alcoholics Anonymous
9:00 am	Physical Education	school ↓	Physical Education	school ↓	Physical Education		↓
10:00 am	Change Clothes 10:15 School Counselor	Lab 10:30-History	Change Clothes Errands	LAB 10:30 - History	Change Clothes Errands	↓	10:30-Lunch
11:00 am	Lab ↓	↓	Lab	↓	Lab	Shopping and Chores	↓
12:00 noon	Logic	Sociology	Logic	Sociology	Logic	↓	Study or Library
1:00 pm	↓ 1:30 - Spanish	↓ 1:30 - English	↓ 1:30 Spanish	↓ 1:30 English	↓ 1:30 - Spanish	Library and Computer time with breaks	and Computer Time with
2:00 pm	↓	↓	↓ Drive Time	↓	↓ Free	as long as needed	breaks
3:00 pm	3:30 - Snack	Study	3:30 - Counsellor	Library	Time ↓		
4:00 pm	Study		Drive Time 4:30 - Free time	↓	Drive Time work		↓
5:00 pm	↓	↓	↓	Drive time		↓	Dinner with a friend
6:00 pm	Dinner Drive	Dinner and Drive time	Dinner	Dinner		Dinner with friends,	6:30 Plan next week
7:00 pm	Study with walking breaks	↓	Study	Study		a movie or hang out	Finish study projects
8:00 pm	↓	Alcoholics Anonymous			↓		
9:00 pm	Watch TV	Drive time					↓
10:00 pm	Bed and Relaxation Time.	Bed and relaxation time	10:30 Bed and relaxation time	10:30 Bed and relaxation time	Bed and relaxation time	10:30 Bed and relaxation time	Bed and relaxation time
11:00 pm							
12:00 midnight							

MONTHLY PLANNER Preferred by a 35 year old male salesman. MONTH Sept.

MONDAY	TUESDAY	WEDNESDAY	THURSDAY	FRIDAY	SATURDAY	SUNDAY
	☺ Dancing	Pay bills		☺ Lunch with mother		yard
	☺ Dancing		Community meeting		~~Work~~	~~Work~~
Work project due	☺ DANCING	PAY bills		prepare work for trip		PACK Leave
Out	of town	→	→	☺ John's 10th b day party		yard
write	☺ DANCING	write	write	Turn in written proposal	DINNER/ Theatre c boss	

5/7 - 5/11

Mon
10:30 Aud.
1p Station
6:30 Aerobics

Tues 9a Hair

Books
2 Good 4 Own Good
BeptD
Wake Up Sleeping Beauty
32 Elephant Kamenko

1p WSRT 600-0000
Call Bob @ Network
6:30p Aerobics

Wed
12n Meeting w/ producer
1p Station
Send card to boss (ratings)

Thurs. 7:30-8 Firestone
8:45 Breakfast
12n P/U car
1p Station

Fri 11:30 Mike J.
1p Station
6:30 Aerobics

Sat 1p John - Hair
Call producer

~~5/28~~
5/14 - 5/21

Mon
1p Station
5p Lee Bennett - Balm

Tues
8:30 Aud.
Call John A @ 611-1111
1p Station

Wed
1p Station

Thurs
1p Station

Fri
1p Station

DAILY ACTIVITY SCHEDULE

NAME:________________________________ DATE:__________________________

DESCRIPTION:____

	MONDAY	TUESDAY	WEDNESDAY	THURSDAY	FRIDAY	SATURDAY	SUNDAY
7:00 am							
8:00 am							
9:00 am							
10:00 am							
11:00 am							
12:00 noon							
1:00 pm							
2:00 pm							
3:00 pm							
4:00 pm							
5:00 pm							
6:00 pm							
7:00 pm							
8:00 pm							
9:00 pm							
10:00 pm							
11:00 pm							
12:00 midnight							

*This form may be duplicated as needed

Step 3: Ask someone to help you. Often, having someone give you a reminder will begin to modify the "On-Off" switch, but only if you have given them permission to do so. Otherwise, they are likely to hit a brick wall.

Step 4: If the person agrees, make a pact that you will practice starting your activity with a reminder from the person.

Step 5: After a reasonable time, ask the person to give you a reminder to stop. Decide on the amount of time beforehand.

Step 6: After some practice with a helper, you can use other devices, such as a timer, to serve as reminders. Eventually, you will have improved to the point that you will be able to overcome the problem simply by thinking about wanting to stop or start at a certain time.

- The "Uh-huh" Phenomenon

Often, people with ADD, when asked something, will say, "Uh-huh" automatically. In reality, they haven't really heard what the speaker said. However, the speaker thinks he or she has been heard and that the person with ADD has agreed to the request or answered in the affirmative. The resulting misunderstanding can sometimes cause problems. To determine if you sometimes do this, ask someone close to you the following question:

"Do I sometimes say 'Uh-huh' but not follow through on the agreement you thought I made?"

If the answer is "yes," it's time to get to work.

Goal: To become aware of saying "Uh-huh" and doing something about the request in a timely manner.

Step 1: Tell the person to whom you say, "Uh-huh" that you want to work on this. Say, "The next time I say 'Uh-huh,' stop me and ask me if I really mean to do what you asked."

Step 2: When the time comes, be honest with your friend. Sometimes, it may be necessary for the person to gently put a hand on either side of your face in order to help you focus on what you are saying.

Step 3: Think carefully if you are really willing to do what the person asks.

Step 4. Consider the consequences of your agreement. You may need to plan ahead in order to honor your agreement.

Step 5: Make a plan for how you will reach the goal in a timely manner.

Step 6: Never agree to anything you don't want to agree to.

- Cutting a Deal

Goal: To gain assistance with tasks you are unable to accomplish. Make a list of everyday living skills that you have, such as mechanical ability, bookkeeping, cooking, or a creative talent.

I can: ____________________ ____________________

____________________ ____________________

____________________ ____________________

List areas in which you need help:

________________ ________________

________________ ________________

________________ ________________

Who do you know who has talent in an area in which you need help?

________________ ________________

________________ ________________

________________ ________________

Ask the person if he would be willing to make a trade with you. Say, "I need help with my bookkeeping." Make an offer to trade one of your skills in return. Say, "I could cook dinner for your family one evening a month in exchange for your help. Would you be interested?"

If you are turned down, ask whether it is because the person doesn't want to do the job or doesn't need what you have offered. If the latter, ask if there is something that the person does need. Say, "Is there something you need that I might be able to supply?" Don't forget to offer money if you have it to trade.

These are only a few of the many exercises that are available to help you with building both your ADD skill base and your ability to do jobs that are hard for you to do because they don't fit your brainstyle. You may need to put yourself through a refresher course every now and again, because the skills don't sit well with your brainstyle. Others, practiced over time, will become habituated, and you'll find you no longer have to think about or accommodate in those areas. You are on your way to making maximum use of your wonderful ADD brain.

7

WORK, DREAMS, AND MAKING A LIVING WITH ADD ATTRIBUTES

The most important job, and one of the hardest jobs in the world, regardless of brainstyle, is finding the job at which you can be both successful and happy.

Finding work is often not easy. Some of you want a safe, secure job with a future, benefits, and guarantees. Some of you want to use your creative dreams, and still others want work that will make the world a better place. There are probably as many agendas as there are individuals. As a result, you have choices to make.

How you go about living *your* life and making your choices is greatly affected by your brainstyle. Your ultimate task is to match the True You to the world in which you live and be able to feel good about yourself and make the living you choose.

How much money you make is not necessarily correlated to your happiness, but the lifestyle you live is. Achieving that lifestyle can be hard if you are a person who has acquired a good case of low self-esteem and poor confidence. Yet you must believe that, with a change in perspective about yourself, you can find your way to happiness in the "job market." Let's start with three common obstacles you and your kindred spirits bump into. Once they are identified, you can do something about removing them.

In typical ADD fashion, let me take a moment to speak about kindred ADD spirits: common to most of us who have an ADD brainstyle is a feeling that we are unique—that awful alone feeling that everyone else is okay, and we're the only ones who are so lost and frightened. I'm here to tell you, you are not alone.

There are lots and lots of us with lots and lots of ADD attributes, and none of us is one of a kind. None of us is a freak, unemployable, or hopeless. We simply have to become familiar with common obstacles we face and learn to negotiate in our ADD way to our goals. We have our own way of doing this—that's what this chapter is about.

COMMON OBSTACLES YOU MAY RUN INTO WHEN SEEKING YOUR PLACE IN THE WORK WORLD

Obstacle 1. Making a living and working may or may not be the same thing, especially if you want to use your dreams and talents on the job. This is what a lot of ADD-style people like to do—even crave to do. Torn between what your heart wants and what your strategic thinking dictates, or what other people say you *should* do, often leaves you feeling confused. But resolving this issue is crucial for you to find happiness. Though it is not easy, neither is it impossible to live your dreams.

Obstacle 2. As you try to fit into traditional ways of being trained for a job and pursue traditional ways to get a job, you're likely to be faced with paperwork and details that are most ADD unfriendly. Training can include reports, outlines, lesson plans, and five-year plans that do not take an ADD brainstyle into account.

Job applications and tests are frequently designed to favor non-ADD applicants. Once you're employed, you may do fine doing the job you were hired to do, but be sunk by needing to keep track of the administrative details that accompany what you accomplish.

There are also the time constraints required by many businesses. If you're the least bit creative or a night person, you may find yourself artificially required to get up, shut down, or prove that you can meet a deadline in a way that doesn't work for you in order to get the job done. For example, if regular reports are required to prove you're progressing toward the goal in a systematic way, you may suffer or even come up short.

Perhaps what you need you'll find hard to get. Let's say it's a need to be left alone to do a job in your own way, even if it means finishing the whole thing at the last minute. Or maybe you need a screen to reduce the chaotic noise and action that surrounds you. When fulfillment of your job-related needs is hard to find, you become discouraged and don't know how to live your dreams.

Obstacle 3. Being in a job that doesn't fit you at all is terrible. It's also much more common than many people think. What if the only job open to you is one that you absolutely can't do adequately, no matter how hard you try? Or you are not allowed to move up to the job you really want, because you are expected to pay your dues doing something that absolutely doesn't fit you. Case in point: Let's say you work for an agency that helps people solve their problems. But you aren't allowed to work directly with the people, helping them solve their problems, until you spend time administering the paperwork needed to acquire the funds for the project, track the progress of each case, and evaluate the outcomes.

WHAT TO DO ABOUT THE COMMON OBSTACLES

First, you must look at the options that are available to you. As you do this, you must realistically consider your situation. Be cautious here. Many folks get very frightened at the thought of not having a job and feel as if they had better take *anything* that comes along. Wrong! Rarely is that a good idea, unless it literally means putting bread on the table for tonight's meal. In that case you are realistically in an emergency situation that requires survival-level living.

Even survival-level living doesn't mean you have to give up your dreams. To be sure, you may need to put your dreams aside for a while, but keep them alive and arduously look for ways to resuscitate them. But let's say you have a little wiggle room. Yes, you need a job, but neither you nor your family is going to starve or end up on the street. You can take the next step toward overcoming the common obstacles you face—a solution that will work for your heart and your pocketbook.

Obstacle 1: Working with your dreams. Thinking outside the box basically means coming up with some ideas for solving your problem(s) that are different from the ones that you've tried before. Ask for help from friends, coworkers, and even people you don't know, but who are successfully doing something similar to what you want to do. Such a person knows the obstacles and the rewards of living from their heart.

Pay attention to the brainstyle characteristics of the person you're asking. Those with an ADD brainstyle are likely to have some ideas that fit your way of doing things. People with a linear brainstyle may mean well, but give you ideas that are unworkable for you. You can tell the difference by listening to your feelings. If you receive an answer that makes your stomach lurch and your mouth go dry, it's probably not one for you to follow up on, despite the idea that "we ought to make ourselves do anything we're afraid of"—an idea held by many people.

I believe fear and hesitation come to you as a gift that can guide you to a path that fits you and away from a direction that doesn't. If the response you receive excites you or makes you feel hopeful, it probably indicates a direction to take, even if you don't know how to proceed. Becoming anxious because you don't know how to reach a goal is totally different from feeling anxious because you don't like what you would have to do to reach the goal.

Technically speaking, asking someone about their job is called information interviewing. It can be done casually or by appointment. Either way, you are not asking for a job—just information.

In the more formal information interview, call the person up and ask, "May I have a few minutes of your time? I'm trying to solve a problem with my work. I know you've been successful, so I wonder if you would be willing to share some of what has worked for you." You certainly can ask how he or she got started. And ask for any tips that will help you be successful.

Sometimes these interviews will be inspiring and extremely helpful. But remember, sometimes they'll fall short when you've not connected with the person who's right for you. I recall once when I was young asking a published writer about getting my first work published. The person was so negative and nonsupportive that I became thoroughly depressed and almost quit before I got started. Luckily, I didn't.

You can also network by asking everyone with whom you come in contact if they know anyone who might talk to you. Soon, you'll have new input and new ideas to pursue.

The next step to fulfilling your heart's desires requires you to realize that *no matter what you like doing, you CAN make a decent living with it*. You may often hear, "Oh, you can't make a living as an artist, musician, or fisherman." But that's not true. The person making the proclamation either doesn't have the skills, interest, or passion to make a living that way, or he or she may have tried but decided to change paths in response to the call of different values, interests, or pressures. The people who succeed as artists, musicians, fishermen, or whatever often have ADD traits. For sure they have an intense desire to work using their special talents and skills. And they are the ones who succeed.

There's also nothing wrong with changing your values. If your desire to make your living as a musician is wearing you out and making you not like music anymore, you may decide to get out of the business. Or perhaps you meet someone you really like and fall in love. The next thing you know, you're going to be a parent. Suddenly, you see things differently than you did before and consciously decide to shift music to what you do to relax and take on a job that both brings in the money and allows some time for your true love, music.

There also isn't anything wrong with deciding to stay with music. Maybe you start to teach music so you can remain in the field but have benefits to boot. A lot will depend upon what you and your partner come to in terms of shared values, interests, and chosen lifestyles. Just be clear about why you're choosing what you're choosing.

Obstacle 2: Organizing your way out of frustration. The most common culprits of organization that are likely to frustrate you are time management, workspace organization, and information storage.

People with lots of ADD characteristics come in two models:

- Multitaskers: those who need to break their jobs into manageable bits. If you're this way, you get more done when you are doing several things at a time.

- "Stick-to-one-thing people." If you're this way, you have to stay with one job until it is completed, because if you take a break, you are likely to fail to return to it.

Pacing helps multitaskers with time management. It's a good idea for you to break each job into small, manageable segments that fit your attention span. Intersperse quiet work with active work. Be sure to give yourself a little reward at break times. Do not wait until the end of the whole task or you'll feel as if you'll never finish and may quit.

When I'm on a deadline—one I want to meet—I have learned to be intensely focused, excluding most day-to-day activities, socializing, and play. I do, however, *have* to take physical breaks or I become depressed. I may weed the garden for a few minutes, swim laps, or do some yoga stretching. I may turn up my music and actively dance.

Physiologically, this gets my juices going, and I can return to sedentary work with renewed vigor until I need another break.

I didn't realize this need when I was in graduate school and spent a lot of time depressed—depression that, in retrospect, could have been avoided if I'd learned to jump rope.

"Stick-to-one-thing people" need to let those around them know not to disturb them. And, if you are this way, you probably will barely want to eat while you're doing something. You won't want to weed the garden, dance, or jump rope. And you don't need to in order to be efficient. You also won't get depressed because of inactivity. You may work late into the night and then catch up on your sleep the next night. Save your reward until the end of the whole task. You'll like it that way.

Your *workspace* may look like it took a kamikaze hit, but if you know where things are, it's okay. The ADD way of organizing requires that things you are working on have to stay out in the open. Once they are filed away, they are "out of sight, out of mind."

Stacks work well. Have a different stack for each project. Use color cues with notebooks, dividers, and paper clips to distinguish one project from another.

Develop a good relationship with your work area in general. It's important to have space to move around. But it is also important to have a separation from others who are working nearby or you're likely to get distracted. Multiple cubicles in a big open area usually don't work for you. You'll probably be very sensitive to noise, so be sure you find a place to get away to do your thinking.

Many a time, I'll say to the members of a team I'm working with, "Excuse me. I need to take this paper outside in order to read it carefully." Nobody cares in the least.

If you're worried about what your boss might think, be up front with him or her. You don't need to wave the ADD banner around as an explanation. Just say, "I want to do a good job for you, so I'm going to take this home to read. I'll have my ideas and answers tomorrow."

Speaking of distractions, sound screens help some people. A radio or even a television can provide white noise, helping to diminish the impact of outside noise. The hum of a ceiling fan or motor can do wonders, too.

There is a lot of information for all of us to gather and store these days. One of the things I noticed early on were two major ways in which people with ADD attributes prefer to keep track of the myriad of details and pieces of information that come our way. One group of people loves, and I do mean loves, to use their computers. Surfing the Internet brings oohs and aahs. Placing addresses and accounting information in your computer is deemed wonderful. Every bit of information is organized by the various software packages that are available. And every bit of information is retrievable.

Then there's the other group of us, who prefer to stay far, far away from computers except as word processors or e-mail tools. For us, interpersonal transfer of information is the best way to obtain and store information. If I receive information from someone directly, I tend to remember it better, couched as it is in the emotions and tenor of the conversation. This includes hard-core facts. Accompany that with a piece of paper with the facts listed, and I've got what I need.

Information sharing for those of you like me means interpersonal sharing. We tend to have interpersonal intelligence. You'll know you're this way if you call someone on the phone or drop by their office before you look the information up on the Internet.

The bottom line in your work environment: allow yourself the freedom to work in the environment that feels best to you. Forget the guidelines generally taught in school or by parents or colleagues. Your intuition is best.

Obstacle 3: The ill-fitting job. What in the world can you do when you are caught in a job that absolutely doesn't fit you? This question is of primary concern because an ill-fitting job is demoralizing, stressful, and terrible for your physical and mental health, much less your happiness and ability to succeed. Happily, you have choices.

The very first thing you must realize is that *good intent is of little value in the workplace.* Conscientious awareness of your weaknesses and the communication of your needs *is* valuable. So what you have to do is stop living on intent, which exists only in the future: "Ah'ma gunna do . . ." Instead, ask yourself, "Do I have a history of being able to do . . . ?" Do not fool yourself into thinking the next time will be different. Have you actually shown (past tense) that you can do it?

Folks with an ADD style of brain construction tend to fall into a trap of "dreaming" (one of our better attributes). I don't want you to curb your dreams; just stop dreaming about what you wish you could do when it comes to your vulnerable areas, which require skills that you don't have. It took me a while to come to grips with this. I do not intend to let myself get in that situation again, now that I've learned, but occasionally I get caught in just plain forgetting that a part of completing a job includes something I have no business dealing with.

A case in point is logistics: the planning and implementation of a delivery system. Recently, I was responsible for getting a children's program into the local schools for fire prevention week. I designed, wrote, illustrated, and piloted the program. I solicited a team member to get the printing bids and make the pickups of the finished material. I contacted the schools to get their involvement. Much to my surprise, I even made a chart listing the participating schools, the number of teachers at each grade level, and the number of kids in each room.

What I forgot were the steps needed to actually use the information on the chart. The packets needed to be sorted for each school ahead of time in preparation for delivery. I also forgot that the boxes of materials would be heavy and needed brawn to carry. I couldn't carry them myself. Nor had I figured how they'd be delivered.

In retrospect, I think I was so impressed that I actually made a chart that it seemed to me that I had "finished" the job. Of course, that was not the case. Logistics! Not my cup of tea. All the good intent in the world does not seem to fill in the blank that my ADD brain simply skips over.

I owned up to my omission, confessing my error to the team leader. I told him I'd misjudged the job and needed help to get the deliveries made on time. I also had a partial solution ready and told him that. I had already asked a coworker to sort the material and make the deliveries. The team leader saw to it that the brawn needed to lift the heavy boxes was available. Then the folks making the deliveries used the chart I'd put together and finished the job.

Sometimes you can clean up your mess by confessing and asking for help. You just can't do it too often. Such confessions and apologies only go so far. I'd already proven my worth to the agency and owned up to the fact I'm no logistics genius. No one on my team expects me to be. But I do need to take responsibility for seeing that I have someone on my team to cover those bases. And I need to not wait until the last minute to do that. I'm working on remembering to plan that piece into every project in which I'm involved.

Never, never try to sweep your error under the rug. And never, ever lie. Doing either of these will surely come back to haunt you. Sometimes, like me, you can clean up your mess by acknowledging your error and asking for help. If you are constantly thrown into the same kind of situation, however, you'll need to go a step further to remedy the problem.

Look around and see if there is some way you can permanently delegate the part of the job that you do poorly. When you approach your boss to change your responsibilities, be sure to have suggestions and solutions at hand. Do not walk in and complain. Instead, make an appointment to present your case.

Be prepared. Start by owning up to your inadequacies. (Remember, everyone has them. The sign of an exemplary employee is that the person knows what he or she can do well.) Then, don't wait for the boss to say "yea" or "nay" to your request. Immediately, present the plan you've worked out ahead of time. It needs to reflect both the way in which the job will or might be done if you don't do it and how you will become more valuable to the company if you are freed from responsibility for what you do poorly. Your plan must take finances into account—all businesses, even nonprofit organizations and agencies, have to deal with a budget.

If your boss doesn't go for your proposal, then you'll have to evaluate how urgent your situation is. You face choices when you are not given the option to permanently rid yourself of the part of your job that you do poorly.

You can make up for some of your weaknesses and vulnerabilities by working extra hard and keeping longer hours. It is at this point that some adults consider medication and training so they can pay more attention to details and perform linear tasks. Either may help you somewhat, but your weak link is still present waiting in the shadows.

Your weak link doesn't mean you're "deficient" or "disordered." Everyone has weak links. No one is good at all steps of a project from the initial vision to creation to implementation to logistics to dealing with the other people involved. You can use aids to help you weather the effects of your weak link; just don't spend much time trying to get rid of that aspect of yourself. For sure, don't trade your strengths in an attempt to overcome your weaknesses.

Set a reasonable period of time to observe the effectiveness of your interventions: no less than three months and no more than six months to tell whether you are going to turn your administration of details around to your satisfaction and to that of your boss. Also evaluate how much stress your interventions place on you.

If you are not satisfied with your performance at the end of your trial period or you do not wish to consider medication and training, you have other options. The first one is to reevaluate yourself and what you really *want* to do. I'm not talking about what you'd like to do, but what you truly want in your heart to be able to do. There's a difference. You may think it would be nice to be thorough and responsible, but that's different from really desiring to do something.

Ask yourself what your goals are. It could be that you wish to explore a different path to your goals, one that does not require you to go through the step(s) that are so likely to cause you major trouble. You may even wish to change your goal(s). You may wish to reinvent yourself. Either way, you have an opportunity to use your creativity to advantage.

REINVENTING YOURSELF

Now you're ready to make strategic moves to reinvent your job or yourself, depending upon what is needed. Let's start with teamwork as a way to satisfy your drives and the demands of a job or business.

Teamwork

If you are working within a company or even if you're self-employed, working as a member of the team may be just what you need. More and more companies are parceling out work dependent upon the skills of their employees. Even major agencies that may not have planned to accommodate brainstyle diversity intuitively fall into patterns that honor the diverse skills of the people they employ.

For example, one major federal agency has two kinds of operatives. Each has the same education and background requirements, but some are made desk agents while others are assigned as field agents. Guess which group has more ADD characteristics. Each is very good at what they do. Each is happy with what they do. If a field agent retires, he or she is more likely to be assigned to training or recruitment than to a desk job with administrative duties.

Generally, a three- or four-member team works well with one person doing details and administration, one visioning, one mo-

Jason's Story: The Middle Path

Forty-two-year-old, matter-of-fact Jason had me stumped. To be sure, he was depressed. He appeared depressed. His wife said so. And he agreed. The problem was that he wasn't responding to antidepressants, psychotherapy, or environmental manipulation.

Several counseling sessions later, I thought about the observations I'd made to date: jiggling foot, constant restlessness during our meetings, and trouble staying on any topic. Add to that his wife's tales of lack of follow-through at home, even at intimate times. He changed jobs often. He'd work for others for a time, become self-employed for a while, get a different job, try a new business, and on and on. Jason also couldn't relax unless he ran, literally, to exhaustion. A marathon runner, he could only fall asleep after his daily training run.

In frustration, I leaned back in my rocking chair, lowered my eyelids, and saw a clear mental picture of nine-year-old Jason confined to a school desk. I saw the same restlessness and watched his agitation grow as he tried to learn in ways that eluded him. He failed to live up to his intelligence, further frustrating his parents, his teachers, and himself.

My mind clicked back into a thinking mode. The first glimmer of what was going on with adult Jason emerged. It just so happened that I was doing a lot of work with adults with Attention Deficit Disorder and, voilà, I realized the probable underlying brainstyle with which Jason was born.

Pairing ADD with his upbringing, I saw clear reasons for his current depression. ADD, in and of itself, is not a reason to be depressed. But when the expectations placed on the growing child are unattainable because of an innate makeup, failure is the only outcome. That's pretty depressing.

I'd already learned that Jason's parents were very concerned that their children be successful. To them, this meant doing well in school, being well-behaved, and working in a traditional job. Jason was "highly socialized." He was taught what successful people look like, how they act, and how they spend their time. The problem was that Jason didn't much fit the model.

His current self-image as a "black sheep" who couldn't achieve had been reinforced for decades. His parents saw him as irresponsible and undisciplined. To make matters worse, they continually bailed him out of scrapes or called in markers to get him into the right college or the right job. More fodder for the low self-esteem mill fed his chronic depression.

Jason never learned who he really is naturally. He didn't learn how to behave or accomplish goals in ways that would fit his brainstyle. He hadn't found anything that made him happy. And he simply didn't know what to do to correct the errors he made, because he was trying to do things that his brainstyle wasn't constructed to do.

(continued)

Viewing Jason's depression and failures in this new context provided new clinical and educational options. The first step was to provide Jason and his wife with information about the effects of his ADD brainstyle. Then he could decide what he wanted to do.

Jason reviewed his work life. With no driving interests or special talents beckoning him, Jason decided his work with computers was acceptable. So, he continued in a field that his parents, too, found acceptable. He also felt more "successful" when he owned his own business. That, too, was a choice that he opted to make.

But because of his brainstyle he made two important modifications. First, he decided he would parcel out some of the organizational and detailed administrative work to someone skilled in that area. His wife, a more naturally linear person, agreed to oversee that aspect of the business. Secondly, he decided to give stimulant medication a try to see if it would help him maintain a focus in the daily running of the company.

Jason also decided to make better use of his natural ADD talents and skills. He offered to spend more time with the kids, ferrying them to their various activities and helping out with schoolwork so that his wife had the time to oversee the business commitment she had agreed to. Jason found he enjoyed coaching the children and listening to their trials, and he found his natural ADD sensitivity worked to advantage. His wife had never much liked that part of the mothering job. She was delighted to get out of the house in order to be around more adults. Jason was delighted to get out of the office to carpool and be a gofer. Everyone won.

Each of them learned more about their styles of brain construction: what they did well and what they didn't do so well. As they each found a higher level of satisfaction, their personal relationship became less contentious. With the new information about brainstyle diversity, their expectations changed. Jason's wife expected different kinds of things from her husband than she had previously—kinds of responses and actions that he could accomplish.

As he was released from trying to do the impossible, his anxiety was reduced and his self-image at finding new interests improved. With tension lowered on the home front, affection began to resurface, and Jason and his wife remembered what attracted them to one another in the first place.

I can only wonder what it would have been like had Jason and his family of origin known about brainstyle diversity and allowed their traditional values to be expressed in ways that fit his particular way of being and doing things. Less pain and stress for Jason and his family would undoubtedly have been the result.

But in lieu of changing the past, the good news is that Jason and his wife gained the opportunity to choose a path with which they could live and were able to pass on to their children what they learned.

tivating and doing public contact work, and one doing hands-on implementation and logistics.

If you can't work as a part of a team, then you may need to take the final step and consider changing jobs. Look at the type of ADD that is dominant for you. (See Weiss, *A.D.D. on the Job*, 1997.) What you are trying to do is match your strengths with the demands of a job. The most important thing to know is how you feel in your heart about a job or particular type of work.

Outwardly Expressed ADD: The Active Entertainer

Typically, people with Outwardly Expressed ADD need opportunities to be expressive, mobile, and outwardly directed. Sales is a natural. You can do retail, wholesale, indoor, or outdoor sales. You can sell products, ideas, concepts, anything.

Maybe you are drawn to being an entrepreneur. Have you always wanted to start your own business? You can be at the cutting edge of something exciting or buy in on a franchise of a more staid business.

Many fields have types of professional jobs at which you could shine. As a lawyer, you might be attracted to flamboyant trial work, or as a physician, emergency room doctoring could be your thing. Teaching, counseling, ministering, and all service work come in all forms: expressive, dramatic, and highly active. Each has its place.

Inwardly Directed ADD: The Restless Dreamer

People with this form of ADD are likely to utilize their creativity and sensitivity. All sorts of art, film, theater, and multimedia projects may be just right for you. Just as outwardly expressive folks do well in teaching, counseling, ministering, and all service work, so too can you if you tend toward Inwardly Directed ADD, only you'll choose a different role to play. Your gentleness and your interpersonal and listening skills work well with people as well as with motors, software, animals, or trees. You have lots of directions to go. Let your interests and desires be your guide.

Highly Structured ADD: The Conscientious Controller

If you have lots of Highly Structured ADD attributes, consider any job that has an inherent structure attached to it. Computer techies, desktop publishers, accountants, and bookkeepers all fall into this category. You can be creative and still be perfectionistic whether you're a home builder who looks at the roofline with your eagle eye or you drive a backhoe cutting trenches with perfection. Whether working as an estate or tax attorney, finding a career in the military, piloting a commercial airliner, or working in any organization that runs in a highly structured way, you will find your niche.

You may blend attributes from more than one of these categories of ADD types—even all three. Sense how you are made and know what you like and what type of job setting you need to fit comfortably into for the rest of your life. With that, you'll find the right spot for you to feel *good* about your job/work life.

TRANSITIONING TO A WELL-FITTING JOB

Making a transition from full-time work that you hate to full-time work that you love may, but doesn't have to, be done in one step. If you come upon a golden egg that buys you time, you can make the step all at once. But if you're like most people, you will need to make the change in smaller increments. It's amazing what you can do after hours when you put your mind to it. Sure beats "vegging," depressed, by the television or drinking too much because you feel so miserable.

Volunteering a little here or there in order to try out interests you have is a good way to begin your transition. Connect with others on the Internet. If you don't have a computer at home, your local library probably has one you can use. At your church, happy hour, children's sport's practices, and everywhere else you go, start talking to the people who are also there. See what other people do. It's not just what a person does to make a living that gives you the opportunity to gather information for your transition. It's what they do when they're not "working." Keep listening and you'll hear of more things than you ever even imagined you might want to do.

I promise you, I never in all my born days thought I'd be working with the Texas Forest Service or any other forest service or natural resource agency. I wouldn't have known to go there to seek a part-time job during my retirement. But I listened when I went to a public meeting about wildfire in the area in which I live. I met firefighters, joined the fire department, met the forest service folks, and over a two-year period learned what they were about. From that, I saw what I could contribute. I also met the people "in charge" and volunteered my help. Next, I voiced my opinion about a few things I observed, and the next thing I knew, the magic words came, "Would you have a few hours to help us modify the direction of our approach to the public?" Seems the natural resource folks know more about handling trees and fire than communicating to homeowners. So I became a contract consultant in a part-time job I love. Well, who would have guessed?

At first, I probably spent only an average of two to three hours a week as a volunteer. It didn't interfere with my other commitments. Later, it grew until I set the limit on the amount of time I wanted to work. Part of where this led me in my transition was to insight that has helped me to become ready to write this edition.

I met a whole different group of people I'd not been in contact with before: rural and small-town citizens. I found many people who have lots of ADD attributes and are living happily and successfully, utilizing their skills and interests in an ADD way.

Living my adult life in big cities and around professionals and academicians, I was limited in my scope of awareness of human diversity. Now I am the richer for living and working where I do. I've also been able through the Texas Forest Service to begin writing for children—a longtime dream. I've even had things published by the agency, so I've gotten a head start on getting my children's work published in bookstore markets. A dream come true! I could not have consciously planned the journey, but I sure recognized the path as it unfolded before me.

Others have followed the same path. You can do it, too. All you need is the belief that you can and the willingness to think broadly, spend your time freely and expansively, and keep your eyes open to the opportunities presented.

An additional benefit is that it feels really good meeting new people and reaching out, no matter what the outcome is. You may even feel that what you are doing in your "day job" isn't so bad after all if your self-esteem is given a boost after hours.

SELF-EMPLOYMENT

Self-employment isn't the way out of the ADD dilemma for everyone, but it sure is for some. Remember, you always have a choice. It doesn't matter if your parents always worked for big companies or your siblings have neither the interest nor courage to become self-employed. If the idea sounds even remotely interesting, explore it. You've nothing to lose as long as you take small steps.

I'm a big believer in trying out a new interest at someone else's expense. Work part-time for a while at a business similar to the one you're thinking about. You'll have an opportunity to see what really goes on in the business. You can see the pitfalls as well as the rewards. Then, if you like what you're doing, you have set yourself up with a high likelihood that you'll succeed.

Times have changed and home-based businesses are proliferating. With computers, you can be anywhere in the world and connect to anywhere else. Many small businesses have emerged in this context.

The rush or high of being in charge of your own business creates a wonderful power trip. You're it, the top dog. That doesn't mean you are a power maniac; it just means that the power and control you have can feel good. Of course, along with power comes lots and lots of responsibility. Ask yourself if you're up for it. If the answer is "yes," you may have found the work style for you.

Whatever dreams your mind imagines, you can attain them. You may buy a secondhand dump truck and haul dirt and gravel and love every minute of your working day. You may opt to work on spec and to design computer programs that you then sell to companies that don't have the money to keep full-time staff on hand to design their own. Perhaps you will choose to buy secondhand stuff, refurbish it, and sell it at flea markets. People make full-time livings doing crafts, writing, catering, and anything else you can imagine. Many of these businesses start small and grow until the owners *have* to quit their full-time jobs to make room for their "other" job.

A few rules of thumb:

- Be sure to have someone keep track of the finances if you aren't good at details. Many a partnership has solved this successfully.

- If your business requires you to work alone, be sure you are good at structuring your time and sticking to a self-made schedule.

- If you're creative, remember that your product has to be sold. Can you do that for yourself, or do you need to hire someone to do sales?

- Many businesses are cyclical. Consider the income averages rather than looking at the highs and lows. Spend accordingly. And have a friend who listens to your fears when the slow-moving times come. It's pretty scary, especially at first.

- As a person with ADD characteristics, the likelihood of your writing an extensive business plan is slim. But you will have to consider coming up with something if you are looking for investors. If you don't have the skill, you'll have to find a trusted financial consultant to do the job for you and advise you about other financial and accounting issues.

- A pleasing personality is crucial and, remember, the client is almost always right. There are ways to avoid taking clients and ways to get rid of customers you don't like, but be thoughtful and skillful in how and when you handle the people with whom you don't want to do business. Blowing up at them or making them angry can bring on a lawsuit at worst or a lot of bad public relations at best.

My experience has shown me that a disproportionately high number of people with an ADD style of brain construction opt for self-employment. Having difficulty making it in the corporate world is not the only reason people turn to self-employment. I think it may be innate. The drive never seems to go away. Even when you're successfully employed by others, with few headaches and great rewards, if the dream to do your own thing persists, you're destined to try your hand at self-employment.

One parting remark I'd like to share with you about self-employment. Though I've occasionally been "employed" by a company or agency, it was usually on contract and not a career job. I just wasn't made to work for someone else. If they expected me to do something that didn't fit me or that I didn't value or believe in, I *had* to say, "no."

I was self-employed as a psychotherapist in private practice and had two children to raise when I got divorced. My dad said, "Well, I guess you'd better go get a real job with a company so you'll have security." I remember how my stomach dropped and my throat constricted so that I could not breathe. It felt as if I were being condemned to prison. I told him "thank you" for the advice and hung up the phone.

Immediately, I realized that there was no way I could take his advice. I also realized that, theoretically, he might be right, but as a self-employed person, I could always work harder to get more business. The power surge I felt with that thought propelled me away from fear and into a feeling of relief. I felt grateful that I could count on myself to do what I needed to do to be successful.

THE CHOICE IS YOURS

There is no one right answer about the right career or job choice for you. The most important thing you must consider is finding the fit between your skills, interests, and desires and the jobs that are available at any given moment.

From time to time, jobs disappear and new ones appear. Printing used to be a viable trade, but was taken over by desktop publishing. On the other hand, the upsurge in computer-related jobs wasn't even imagined thirty years ago. Nothing stays the same.

One year, you'll hear how there aren't enough teachers. A few years later, there will be too many teachers. Or one locale will have too many and another will have too few. One job category will pay well at one time, only to be surpassed by another job category a decade later. Sometimes when you start an educational program, you'll think you've got everything figured out, career-wise, only to find out later that you are doing something totally different than you ever guessed you'd be doing.

Flexibility and the willingness to change are the key. Always have a plan B or at least the awareness that the time may come when a plan B is needed and the willingness to construct it.

Be prepared to make trades for what you want. If you need stability, you may trade that for a higher income. Or if you need the freedom to change, get bored once you learn something, and hate repetition, you also may need to trade freedom and mobility for a high income or job security. Just know the potential price you may need to pay to get what you want—and I don't just mean the dollar value.

Most of us live long enough to engage in more than one career. Often we have several. There's time in our lives to live out most of our dreams. We just can't live them all at the same time. When you've small children at home, you may not want to be moving constantly or working long hours. On the other hand when you're older you may want to travel, see the sights, and meet new people. Your circumstances will shape the kind of job you seek.

There is simply no one rule of thumb about employment, jobs, or moneymaking. Be who you are, lighten up, and let your imagination be your guide. There is simply no reason to remain in a job that you hate or that makes you feel like a failure. If you are in a setting where your performance makes you the boss's scapegoat, no amount of training or medication will help. You must consider other options. Take your courage in hand and believe enough in yourself to know that you and everyone else have value. You just have to find the place you'll be appreciated and the kind of work that makes you feel happy and proud of yourself.

WORKING WITH AN ADD PERSON

Whether you are the person with a number of ADD attributes or you work with someone who has them, you will need to be sensitive to the effects of the characteristics on others and on your work relationship. Coworkers and bosses are likely candidates requiring you to make adjustments in your thinking and your approach to your job because of the brainstyles involved.

When you came for the job interview and met your new coworkers, there may have been few signs identifying who had what brainstyle. But day in and day out, working with someone with unrecognized and unaccommodated ADD has led to frustration, lost motivation, and feelings of resentment over having to do more than your fair share. And the worst part is that, unlike home, where you can blow off steam with your spouse, child, or parent, on the job you have to deal with the problem and your feelings about it without openly acknowledging that they even exist. You have to take responsibility for managing their ADD and yours, if you are also ADD.

Common Questions about Work, Dreams, and Making a Living

The following common questions and their answers will help you learn what you can do to make life easier on the job when you work with or for someone who has ADD but is not taking responsibility for it. These examples are taken from real-life situations with real people who have either been identified to have ADD or who believe they are working with someone with unrecognized ADD.

My boss agrees to my plans one day and the next day tells me he never said "yes." How can he not remember what he said?

Typical of ADD is a phenomenon in which the person says, "yes" automatically without fully digesting the request being asked. Sometimes it's in order to be the "good guy." Sometimes, the person is thinking about something else, but is acknowledging your presence without contributing enough attention to your question to follow through.

Your job is to confirm that the person hears you. You can do this by reiterating what you believe was agreed upon. Then say, "What time tomorrow shall we follow up on this?"

My coworker has all sorts of ideas but doesn't follow through on any of them. Is she just irresponsible?

Could be, but maybe not. Could be that her intent is to follow through but she takes on more than she can manage. Or maybe she gets distracted by something else that intervenes. Maybe she doesn't know how to set limits on others' requests.

To be honest with you, most people who appear irresponsible are trying the best they can. There could be all kinds of reasons why they don't follow through, from emotional problems to being overwhelmed with daily activities to not processing auditory requests efficiently.

To protect yourself, don't depend on someone for something if that person has repeatedly let you down. Watch to see what the person *can* be counted on to do, and then don't keep expecting more than that. Don't spend your time when the other person says, "I'd like to do . . ." or "Hey, I have a great idea." Have the person take the next step to begin the project and then commit a small amount of time before he or she takes another step.

My boss jumps from one topic to the next without resolving any of them. Business meetings seem pointless, but I can't refuse to attend. What can I do?

You can take a pad and do your own work during the meeting.

From time to time, you can suggest to your boss that you skip a meeting to complete a project.

You can ask pointed questions during the meeting so that you get what you need out of it.

You can listen to the topics your boss raises during the meeting, identify the ones that pertain directly to you, and after the meeting, go to the people from whom you need input and get it personally rather than in the group. If you need further input from your boss, you might try to get it in writing or by e-mail.

Whenever I have something long or complicated to explain to my boss, he doesn't seem to be able to focus on what I'm saying. How can I communicate with him more effectively?

Try putting what you have to say in written form. Maybe even outline it. Give him direct written questions to answer with "yes" or "no" answers.

If you talk with him, give him one question at a time. Get the answer to that one before going on to the next questions. Don't expect to have lengthy conversations. Rather, touch base with him several times during the day so that your encounters are broken into small segments. Do the same with e-mails. One topic per e-mail may work a lot better than ten topics in one e-mail.

My boss can't seem to remember a production schedule she has worked with for years. Is she just not trying?

It's possible she doesn't care and isn't trying, but it's not likely. After all, it is her living also that's in jeopardy.

Unless she has a chemical abuse problem, head injury, or chronic life stress, she probably simply does not think about schedules, especially if she is a creative type of person. She may also get distracted by all sorts of issues that emerge in the daily running of a business or by her own ideas.

Your best bet to remedy the problem is to help her out by creating and posting a schedule that you remind her about regularly. She is likely to feel very grateful. Take as much personal responsibility as you can manage to keep up with it. Use her skills where they shine.

My boss is rigid and gets very upset if I deviate one little bit from the schedule he insists we use.

Here's the flip side of the above coin. This boss has either compensated for his organizational deficits by rigidly adhering to a schedule or has many of the attributes of Highly Structured ADD. If he gets off schedule even a little bit, he'll get off a lot. There tends to be no middle ground.

You can try talking to your boss. Explain that your way of working is different from his. Point out that you get your job done on time and at a high level of quality. Ask if he can trust that you will continue to produce adequately.

The problem, though, may not be his lack of trust in you but his inability to maintain organization if everything isn't slotted perfectly, as he would do it. If this is the case, you may need to consider working for someone else.

The guy I work with just seems to bounce around. He has so much energy that he's like a puppy. How can I calm him down?

There may be little that you can do to calm him down. Though most people who have an ADD style of brain construction have increased motor activity, only some have hyperactivity that is as noticeable as your coworker's. You can talk and move smoothly and soothingly. Your manner can calm him down a little. You may be able to affect him if you simply talk in a slower manner. Lower your voice.

Hopefully, your coworker is not tied to a desk and has reasons to move around, preferably outside, at least some of the time.

Send him on errands and give him reasons to get up and do things for you. Or walk with him, talking as you move. He will be grateful for the opportunity to move around.

Everyone likes our public relations director because she is so creative, cheerful, and friendly. But she just doesn't get her work done on time and holds up the production process. I'm the one who has to follow through for her, but if I confront her I'm viewed as the bad guy. Is there any way to win in this situation?

Be very straightforward with her. But also be empathetic. She does need to do something about her lack of follow-through. Tell her honestly about the problem you face because she doesn't have her material on time. Ask her for possible solutions. If she gives you some, try them out. If she doesn't, say, "I know you're doing the best you can and I like you a lot, but I can't run short again next week. Is there anything I can do to help you?" Offer help, but don't set yourself up as a judge.

If there continues to be a problem, ask her to join you for a discussion with your boss to work out a solution. That way you don't have to be the bad guy, and you can get what you both need. Remember, this need not be a win-lose situation. It should be a win-win one.

If you're empathetic with her, you may be amazed at how she brings her fears and problems to you, considering you a friend.

I hired a woman I thought was wonderful, but she can't ever finish what she starts. My coworkers expect me to handle the work—she's my employee, after all. But if I say something to her about her lack of follow-through, she says I'm picking on her. What can I say to make things better? What are my options?

The way in which you bring her attention to her inadequacies is important. If you tell her what's wrong without telling her how to fix it, she will feel helpless. After all, if she could have done it right in the first place, she would have. Instead, point out what you like or find acceptable in her work. Do this in a matter-of-fact way. Then show her how to apply that to something else she is doing.

Be sure to give her small assignments that are very specific. You may be giving her too much at one time so she can't focus. Give her breaking points in the work so she can naturally change her focus rather than have her lose focus. What I'm talking about is providing more structure. (The military does this effectively.)

If your employee has an attitude problem, you can mention it to her, asking whether something is bothering her personally—something she has been unable to leave at home.

Then, remember, if you hired her, you can fire her. You can do it humanely by taking responsibility. Say, "I made a mistake and hired you to do something that doesn't fit your capabilities. The job is not getting done, and you aren't getting the satisfaction of doing a job well."

You may want to counsel her with regard to a job that would better suit her. Or maybe you've come to realize that she's depressed, in which case you might suggest she seek help with her feelings so she can feel better. Refer her to an outplacement counselor or support group that can work with her attentional issues and emotions.

If she still insists you are picking on her, say, "I'm sorry you feel that way, but it seems I can't do anything to make things better." Then back off. Hopefully, you've kept records of her behavior and your attempts to work with the situation, so you can back up any retaliatory action she might take when you let her go.

The husband of one of my best employees is a salesman. She is often late to functions, saying, "My husband just can't get anywhere on time." What could be the problem? What can she do to correct it?

There are many reasons people are late. ADD is one, but by no means the only one. It could be his way of asserting his power in the relationship. It could be an expression of the fact that he doesn't want to go.

What she can do to correct it is take responsibility for getting herself to the function on time. She can come ahead, and her husband can join her later. How she works that out with him is her business. You just keep the limit in place that you expect her on time, and don't let her use her husband as an excuse.

My boss changes his mind about our plans all the time. He seems to jump from one idea to another. It causes me to make a lot of false starts, wastes a lot of my time, and makes me feel frustrated. How should I talk with him about this, and will it do any good?

Go to him and say you appreciate the many ideas he has. Say, "But I'm the kind of person who needs to follow through on an idea, and that's why you hired me. I need you to choose which idea you want me to work on to completion." Speak in a firm, slightly serious but warm manner. This lets him know you mean business but are not being critical.

When he again starts spewing off new ideas, make a list of them, and show him the list, along with a list of the projects you are already involved with. Ask him to set priorities. Say, warmly and firmly, "Remember, I need to feel good about finishing something." That way, the burden is placed on him with regard to how you spend your time.

Most creative people, with or without ADD attributes, appreciate having someone like you around. Your boss needs you desperately but just doesn't know how to use you. Help him learn.

My boss only seems to want to dream and make big plans. I'm beginning to think she does this because of the excitement she gets out of it. Could that be?

Sure could. There is a high (an adrenaline rush) that comes from the making of big plans. Some people get it from just having a wonderful idea. The feeling that comes from the high is so good that the person tends to want to feel it again and again. Once the feeling has passed, there is little interest in continuing to develop the plan. After all, it's pretty hard to get a rush from following up on mundane details, especially if you are a creative person. Sometimes the person doesn't know how to follow up.

Our sales manager can't seem to organize his own time. I see this in other sales reps also, so I'm not sure I'll do much better if I fire him. Besides, he makes good sales. Any suggestions?

There is a higher than average number of people with ADD who are drawn to sales positions. They often do very well. However, organization, at least in a linear way, is frequently not their strong suit.

First of all, if your salesman is doing a good job selling, rather than being critical, consider applauding him. Also, his way of organizing may simply be different from yours. If he's making the sales, he must be organizing adequately to get the job done.

In addition, keep paperwork to a minimum. Try providing simple, clearly structured report sheets. Have the person take part in the development of the reporting forms.

Break reporting tasks into small segments. For example, have the salesman report daily instead of weekly. When he's on the road, have him fax or e-mail the reports back to the office every day.

Empathize and use humor with your errant salesperson and be grateful for what you do have.

Consider hiring a clerk so your salespeople only have to collect raw data that someone else puts in boxes. Then the salesperson can sell more to pay for the clerk.

8

RELATIONSHIPS AND ADD

PARENTING AND ADD

My heart goes out to parents who are frustrated beyond words, trying to *get* their offspring to act responsibly.

My heart goes out to the adult children who didn't learn to be responsible when they were younger.

No one is to *blame.* This is an equal opportunity problem. With a child who has struggled in school or sometimes has problems with other kids, it's very easy for parents to give in. The result is that a child who grows into adulthood without having learned to be responsible becomes an irresponsible adult.

Not withstanding, as the adult, *you* have as much responsibility as your parents to take hold of your life and make use of the wonderful potential with which you were born. And you have the responsibility to learn to curb the bad habits that plague you. An approach that I am going to take in this section is to let you look over your parents' shoulders as I outline what needs to happen to right the wrong so you can move forward. I want your parents to realize that they had to "pick their battles." Some of the reasons for the problems you faced were learned and a lot may not have been.

Sometimes the expectation is that when a young person reaches eighteen, he or she will automatically know what to do to live responsibly. But that's not how it works. Learning to be responsible is a slow process learned a step at a time. It won't take eighteen years as a young adult to learn the skills, but it may take several. Accumulating experiences that do the teaching is what takes the time. This means amassing both failures as well as successes.

Without realizing it, we parents usually assume that our children will be "chips off the old block." This means that our kids will want what we want, learn the way we learn, and dream the same dreams we dream. Unfortunately, that's not necessarily so! We may not have had the kind of child we expected or wanted. This is as true of biological children as of adopted kids.

This doesn't mean we parents don't love all our offspring. We do. It's just that some are easier for us to understand and respond to than others. By the way, the same is true in reverse. Some parents are easier for kids to live with and learn from than others, for all the same reasons. Often, we are more comfortable with people who are more like ourselves, and we don't know what to do with differences.

There are many cultural and social standards that do not take diversity into account and that may make our children *seem* to be "problems." A parent may have encountered endless challenges in school settings with a youngster who learned in a style that was not the reward-gathering, popular way. Of course, the ADD child had no clue what to do about his or her school situation, either, so lost children are being led by lost parents. The usual result is a child who's labeled a behavior problem. Add to all this the fact that children with ADD may not learn the way they were taught—and that includes how they were taught by the parent.

As a parent, you may not have known about ADD until recently or about the abuse piled up over the years on the shoulders of your child. Please do not feel guilty. You have lots of company. So few people knew, or know, about ADD that even today you cannot feel responsible for problems that have built up. But they did build up, layer upon layer.

Both parents and children did the best they could. But realize any adult child will need help to overcome the repercussions of abuse and lack of useful training. Remember, the young adult *and* the parents must work together to turn the situation around.

What you can do, however, is start today.

1. Sit down together and assess the situation of the young adult. You may wish to use an outside counselor or mediator to help with this if the relationship leaves a lot to be desired, with anger and resentment running rampant. To accomplish step 1, the following must occur:

   - If drugs or alcohol or other addictive behavior is involved, that must be faced up to immediately before any partnership work can occur.

   - Parents must leave their guilt behind and become clear-headed about their role as parents.

- Both parents and adult children must leave their anger behind and be willing to deal as equals who have different skills. No one is in charge, nor can anyone make the other do anything.

- Adult children must let bygones be bygones and accept the fact that their parents did what they thought was best—even when it was totally wrong.

- Parents must also let bygones be bygones and accept the fact that their children did what they knew to do—even when it was totally wrong.

- Adult children must be willing to honestly face their fears and work to change their situations rather than expect to live the way they were under their parents' roof.

- Parents must walk the fine line between rescuing their adult children and giving them only what they truly need to make the next step.

- Both parents and adult children need to remember that growing up is a process, not an event.

2. Parents, you can intervene with the outside world on behalf of the young ADD adult as much as is needed but slowly do less and less.

3. Parents, you must give your young adult children increasing responsibility with each month and year and let them know you believe they will succeed. When failure occurs, focus on what can be learned to avoid the same failure in the future rather than wringing hands or scolding or shaming your son or daughter.

And you, young adults, must "get right back on the horse" and try again with some new information under your belt and new strategies or adjusted values that up the odds you'll succeed the next time. No feeling sorry for yourself or dulling the pain of failure with anything that gets in the way of your next success.

Maybe you don't succeed to the degree you've dreamed about—after all your ADD sensitivity and big-picture enthusiasm make for pretty big dreams—but you still can go on. Scale down and take a smaller step next time. You don't need the enemy of impatience hounding you. One step leads to the next, to the next, and to the other side of the river!

4. Parents, if your adult child doesn't work constructively with a failure, you must not enable him or her. For example, let's say you already helped your adult child clear up some outstanding traffic tickets. You thought she'd learned her lesson but she recently received a number of others that have not yet been paid. There's a warrant out for her arrest. This time, do not run in to pay them so she won't be arrested. That would be enabling.

   You may go with your daughter to court, but not pay her fines. Instead, become firm. This could mean going to Alanon, a counterpart to Alcoholics Anonymous for family members and friends of alcoholics, if she is an alcoholic, or it could mean seeing a counselor or getting your neighbor to hold your hand while you maintain the limits you have set for your daughter.

5. Parents, let go of *your* dreams for your son or daughter, potential and all. Instead, you can help him or her uncover

his or her own dreams. Listen well. Then support the dreams to the best of your ability.

At the same time, sons and daughters, listen to your heart and imagine what you'd like to do. Don't be afraid to dream. Then ask for advice on how to reach your dreams.

Sons and daughters need to work just as hard at achieving their dreams as parents work for them. If you as a parent did not pursue your own dreams, you are in danger of trying to push your adult children to live out theirs *and* yours together. This approach will backfire. Instead, serve as a model to your kids by pursuing your own dreams. It's never too late.

6. Parents, let your ADD young adult follow a creative path toward adulthood if he or she wishes. Just because everyone else in the family earned a college degree right after high school doesn't mean your child has to want one, too. I'm not saying a person with ADD can't make it in college, but that the decision needs to be made by the individual.

   If you, as a young adult, are the one desiring to pursue a creative path, all you have to do is be responsible in that pursuit. This means learning and developing your skills, spending plenty of time pursuing ways to make headway using your creativity, and asking for some help, but not expecting others to totally support you.

   Be wary. Talking about your dreams is not the same as working to accomplish your dreams. You may have to get part-time work to support yourself, for as an adult, you are responsible for your livelihood. You won't be the first to have a day job while you go after your dream job.

7. Parents, you need to communicate a belief in your young adult's ability to do well, including making a living. This is simply a matter-of-fact circumstance of life—self-support. If your child whines or says that "creative people" are so sensitive that they can't be expected to work like everyday people, just shrug and say, "Well, here you have to work, too."

   Parents, do not be pressured or get into an argument if pushed. If your offspring tries to keep up the argument, tell her to leave. She's on her own. By the way, such dysfunctional behavior may be a sign of drug or alcohol abuse. I suggest getting yourself to Alanon immediately.

   Above all, no "enabling." Some support, especially financial, is fine, but don't let it become a habit. If you recycle the same problems and the same outcome, you need as parents to turn responsibility for the problem over to your adult child. No ifs, ands, or buts. And remember, slow steps toward your young adult taking more and more responsibility and providing self-support little by little is crucial.

   Young adults, you need to let parents know when you stumble or run into disappointments. This doesn't mean whining about the bumps and bruises.

   You can expect a hug or pat on the back, maybe a special dinner and some well-meaning advice, but then you'll need to get right back up, just like when you were little, and keep on going.

8. This last guideline is a hard-and-fast rule: if the young adult begins acting irresponsibly or destructively, let him

or her take responsibility for the repercussions of his or her actions.

And if you're the one who is getting out of control, the most important thing for you to do is get support and direction from people who won't enable you to stay irresponsible and destructive. This could take the form of going to Alcoholics Anonymous (AA) or Narcotics Anonymous (NA) or getting some career counseling.

I'm really tough on this issue. Let natural consequences happen, even if it means jail time for criminal behavior, driving-under-the-influence arrests, or missing important appointments because of staying up too late partying the night before. A parent can offer to help an adult child get help. An adult child can ask for advice, but must not expect a parent to bail him or her out. Separation may end up being the only way possible until parents stop overparenting or sons or daughters stop acting like little, out-of-control children.

ADULT SIBLINGS AND ADD

As we all know, brothers and sisters can be the best of friends and the worst of enemies. Sometimes, this changes from minute to minute. Sometimes, siblings get stuck in one position or another. And all too often, ADD will play a role in problems between them.

When ADD goes unrecognized in childhood, the frustration and difficulties associated with mishandled ADD build up. The kid with a lot of ADD attributes may become the "bad" kid, and the one who does things in a more acceptable, linear fashion may be labeled the "good kid." If this problem goes on long enough, it can blind the adults to what is really going on.

The best way to handle this is to be matter-of-fact about the new information being gained with respect to having an ADD brainstyle. Parents and siblings can speak in terms of brainstyle diversity. This takes judgment out of the communication, and that's imperative. After all, each sibling will have strengths and weaknesses, no matter how they appear on the surface. Once the differences are recognized for what they are—differences—the worst of the battle is over.

It's very important, if this applies in your situation, that neither you nor your sibling place blame. As the one with lots of ADD characteristics, you have had and may still have a plateful of difficulties if your family didn't know how to handle things. So it's time to share what you are learning about both taking advantage of what your attributes can do for you and owning up to some of the problems that occur because you don't know what to do about the way you are made.

You don't have to apologize, but you do have to try see the difficulties faced by your sibling(s) because of your brain construction. For example, it's possible that your folks had to spend so much time helping you that others were overlooked and their needs didn't get met. Or maybe your frustration got the best of you, and you took it out on your brother or sister. Maybe you were the one who was made responsible for all of you getting punished because you didn't do your part of the chores. Own up to some typical issues and your adult siblings will begin to feel more understood. And when they feel more understood, you'll be looked upon more kindly.

If you're the sibling who was the "good" one or who came up with the short end of the stick because of your brother's or sister's ADD issues, you may feel a range of emotions, from not wanting to lose your preferred status to being very angry. I'd ask you: "Why in the world would that make a difference? You know what you're made of. You're no longer a child seeking parental approval. You are an adult and have the ability within yourself to approve or disapprove of yourself. Be honest. Appreciate what you've done that you're proud of. Work harder on anything that pleases you or that you want to develop but find hard to do."

If you're still resentful of what happened when you were a kid, ask yourself why. Consider a talk with your ADD sibling to get the other side of the story. Then, with a fuller picture, see how both of you were hurt or shortchanged.

Being denied a sibling's favor and approval is tough. Learning to be compassionate and understanding is a real gift you can give, and one that you can receive in return. If you find this a hard task to handle, get some family counseling, and you'll be mighty glad.

Personality differences will always be a factor. Brainstyle differences will always have to be bridged. But the potential for camaraderie and teamwork make up for the price of the work involved. The end result may even allow love to blossom in a way that it never could before.

LIVING IN A COMMITTED RELATIONSHIP

Living in a committed relationship takes lots of understanding by both parties. Although people with a predominantly ADD style of brain construction are often singled out as "the problem," any two people trying to make a go of living together will confront differences in how they do things and what they think is important. You are no more responsible for the problems than the other person.

Always remember that your brainstyle is one of the reasons your partner was attracted to you in the first place. To be sure, brainstyle differences work no differently than any other differences. Whatever attracts us to our partners and friends is also what eventually causes us the most trouble.

Okay, philosophy aside, your partner's ADD attributes may add zest to your life, creativity to your world, and sensitivity and feelings to your psyche. That doesn't mean that your partner folds the laundry the way you like. (Yes, this example is from a marriage counseling session I once led.) Getting to places on time, keeping a neat house, or managing the family finances may not be a part of your wonderful ADD partner's skill base. But, I promise you, someone who manages the books, is always on time, and keeps a neat house may not be nearly so much fun to live with. It's important to pick your battles and be realistic about your expectations.

Here are some tips to help you and your ADD partner live in peace, acceptance, and respect.

- No matter what your brainstyle, know that there are things you can improve about yourself and things that will not change. Be accepting of both. Do all you can do to improve your livability, but do not expect that you'll be any more well-rounded than most other people.

- Leave judgments out of the picture. Often the partner who has few ADD attributes thinks of himself or herself as the one in the right. This is especially true if the person keeps a neat house, is timely, and is good about follow-through. Those are, after all, cultural values that are considered next to godliness. Instead, remember, they are only values that are entrenched in the Western culture as significant. Not all cultures believe this way. Not all families put these values ahead of others, such as the communication of warmth, the sharing of feelings, and the pursuit of a creative or playful lifestyle.

- Separately list your strengths and weaknesses. Own them and consider which ones you'd like to change. Then set priorities for changing them. Be realistic. After several tries at changing something, you may need to reconsider the probability of changing it anytime in the near future. (The odds that I'll never burn a pot again while cooking are mighty low, no matter how hard I try to remember to turn it off, even when I set a timer. That's just reality. I'm sure not beating myself up about it, and neither would I let someone else shame or criticize me because of it.)

- Once you've done your own individual work, share what you've come to with your living partner.

- Next, share what bothers each of you about the other. Again, no blaming or shaming. You're only listing facts. You must realize that each partner is currently doing the best that he or she can do. A commitment to change can come in the future, and even then, you don't know if it will be realistic or not. Maybe it will. Maybe it won't.

Living with someone takes lots of understanding on both sides, much ability to trust in one another's best intentions, and lots of negotiation skills. As long as each person is good of heart, reasonably mentally healthy, and willing to take responsibility and let the partner work on himself or herself, the relationship has a good prognosis.

If one person needs to be over-controlling or particularly needs to keep the person with lots of ADD attributes inadequate, then a healthy relationship is unlikely. In fact, if you are the one who is working on improving your livability, you are likely to gain less favor as you improve than you had when you were more inept. This same pattern is seen with recovering alcoholics. The "good" partner only feels comfortable and safe as the "better" partner. This is not a healthy relationship.

Quality relationships can survive—and flourish—when there are two winners and no losers. This takes seeing the other's point of view, communicating an understanding of that viewpoint, and seeking a resolution to issues until a mutually suitable solution is found—one that you both can live with. Good luck and keep at it until you find the answers.

TIPS FOR LIVING EFFECTIVELY TOGETHER

Negotiation

Blaming can be such a large part of an ADD person's life—and the lives of those who live with them—that learning negotiating skills is not only desirable but necessary as well.

Whether you are a spouse, partner, friend, parent, colleague, or person with lots of ADD attributes, follow these guidelines and you may be surprised at how well they work.

- You must accept that it doesn't matter why something happened. Placing blame is of no value.
- It does matter *what* happened.
- Eliminate all judgment from your discussion. (Later, you can work on eliminating judgment from your thoughts, too.)

- Get to the facts without lots of excuses, apologies, or stories.

- Each partner needs to come up with a plan to solve the problem. Keep them simple.

- Communicate your general plan to your partner and listen to his or her plan. When you're sharing your plan, your partner needs to refrain from interrupting you. It's all right to ask questions for clarification after the plan has been shared. You must similarly restrict your comments when your partner is sharing.

- Each partner then says what he or she likes about the other's plan. Also say what will need to be modified, but be sure not to judge or criticize any part of the plan.

- Modify each suggested plan, set priorities, and tell your partner what is very important to you.

- Merge your plans so you have one focus.

- Work on only one thing at a time.

- Together lay out specific ways to accomplish the steps in your plan that are mutually acceptable.

- Set the plan in motion, one step at a time, and stick to it unless you both sit down and renegotiate a new plan. You'll get used to negotiating your needs, and you will end up feeling like, and being, a winning team in the long run.

Follow-through can be a problem, especially for people with a lot of ADD attributes. Distractions may get in the way, having the effect of pulling you off course.

In relationships, lack of follow-through destroys trust. Rarely does an ADD person mean to hurt anyone. But the effect can be one of hurt.

Your partner needs to not take lack of follow-through personally. It's not lack of caring and love.

As an ADD-prone person who's easily drawn off course, take on only what you truly *want* to do. Avoid doing something because you think you *should*.

Partners of ADD folks, you must not automatically assume it is your right to issue reminders to your errant ADD partner. The person with the ADD attributes must ask you to extend a reminder. If you're willing, it can be helpful during the learning stage. It takes time for new behaviors to become habit. You can both think of it as practice time to help your ADD partner to learn to follow through.

The person you ask doesn't *have* to take on the responsibility. Sometimes, partners are pretty angry and fed up with what they perceive as their carrying "all the responsibility." That's rarely the total truth, but a deteriorating relationship can become much like a parent-child relationship. In that case, asking the tired, angry partner for help may not work well.

It is, however, a nice thing to do, but it's better for the person with the ADD attributes to do the asking than for the non-ADD person do the offering.

Bear in mind that lists and schedules can be the ADD person's best friend. Requesting help to construct them is fine. Keeping them up-to-date probably means a non-ADD person will have to give a helping hand. Even better, both people could go over the lists together. That's good training, and the carrying of joint responsibility can bring togetherness. If you fight over the lists or get into a scolding, excuse-making match, forget about working together.

Sensitivity

Thin skin is a major attribute of Attention Deficit Disorder. The more ADD attributes, the more likely you are to have thin skin. What this means for you is that you can be easily hurt or offended. It also means that you'll respond by either lashing out or imploding—that is, getting depressed or becoming stubborn. None of these responses is very useful when you are in a meaningful relationship.

When the partner who doesn't have a lot of ADD attributes says sharply, "Quick, we're late. I just looked at my watch, and we're already late," you are likely to resist or become irritated. The more you're prodded, forced, or yelled at, the more likely you will resist. Better to respond with, "Your pushing me isn't helping. I'll hurry the best I can." Or say, "You go on ahead. I'll meet you there."

When the pressure is on, it is no time to try to talk through this problem. Instead, prepare ahead of time. You can agree to go separately when you're running late. You can ask your partner to remind you to get going, say an hour ahead. Then, of course, it's up to you to get going. You can develop a cue you both understand, such as holding your hand up with your palm facing the frustrated person and saying, "Whoa, slow down, and I'll hurry up."

Cutting a Deal

Lack of follow-through affects both participants in a relationship. It's tough to be the one who lets another down. And it's tough to be let down. It tends to create a parent-child type of relationship, usually with the ADD person taking on the role of the child and the partner becoming the parent. Not good!

Rarely does either person mean to hurt the other—except once anger has built up. Under these conditions, trust becomes damaged or destroyed, requiring major remediation if the relationship is to be spared. It's better to minimize the damage by cutting a deal ahead of time.

- Tell your partner that you're working on improving your skills (timeliness, follow-through, etc.). This, of course, means you are truly committed to learning new ways to be responsible and don't just put your partner off. No more throwing your hands up in the air, giving up, or denying that you have a problem that needs attention. And no blaming the other person for expecting too much.

- Ask for reminders, saying you really intend to follow through but tend to get off track, to over-schedule, and to under-organize.

- Take extra responsibility to remind yourself. For example, if you are more responsible at work than you are at home, where you tend to let down, you may add personal items to your appointment book. After all, you're used to looking at it as work, so you're halfway there. Try mounting a sign on your refrigerator. Do whatever it takes to become self-responsible. Lists and schedules may be your best friends.

- From time to time, especially when you're tired, you are likely to relapse. Tell your partner this and reaffirm that a reminder would be mighty nice.

- Don't forget to apologize when you "goof up," but don't apologize constantly without changing, in order to try to improve the current situation.

- It's important to agree only to what you want to do. With your sensitivity, it's difficult for you to fake it effectively. You need to be honest.

COMMON QUESTIONS FROM FRIENDS AND FAMILY MEMBERS

I feel very guilty about what we did and allowed to be done to our son when he was a child. Is there anything we can do to feel better? And what can we do for our son?

For yourself, please be forgiving. Know that you did the very best you could do at the moment you were doing it. Had you known a better way, you'd have used it.

For your son, sit down with him and tell him of your new awareness. Give him information. Tell him you think he did a tremendous job surviving thus far and that you would like to support him. And you might want to help him get some relearning if he would like to. There's nothing wrong with including financial support for school or retraining, if he requests it or accepts your offer accompanied with a plan and follow-through.

Don't overdo to make up for the past. Don't take responsibility to fix him now because you feel guilty. Rather, form a partnership with him in which he does all he can do, and you help out where you can. You may want a counselor to help you determine where the line between helping and enabling lies.

Why does my ADD husband get all his jobs done at work and fail to get anything finished at home? He's either a couch potato watching TV or he's sleeping.

It's not unusual for adults with ADD to use up all their energy focusing their attention at work. By the time they get home, there's no energy left for goal-directed behavior.

Don't take his behavior personally or think he doesn't care. Talk with him about setting aside a specific time, after a rest, to do one thing at a time. Let him know it would really help you.

It also might be a great help to do some of the chores together. Teamwork often is effective in helping the ADD person stay centered on an activity.

From the sound of things, my non-diagnosed adult with ADD son married a non-diagnosed adult with ADD woman. I've never understood how they can have such verbal uproars and then make up after a little while. What can they do?

Very possibly their uproars bother you more than them. Theirs is a common pattern when two people with ADD find each other. It's wonderful or awful. But remember they probably understand each other on a very deep level, because of their shared brainstyle. They would both benefit, though, from some training to find other ways to communicate that might be less emotionally charged. It would be especially useful if they decide to have children.

Why is it better the person with ADD makes up a reminder list?

Because a person with ADD feels everything acutely, he does better when he's in control of what affects him. Making up that list puts the power and responsibility in the right hands. It's also good training for him.

How do I "depersonalize" my experience trying to negotiate with someone who's ADD?

Use your brain instead of your feelings.

Think about what is happening.

Think about what you would like to happen.

Be aware of what you're feeling: fear, frustration, helplessness.

Take responsibility for your feelings and learn what you need to do in order to attend to them.

Even though I understand a lot more about ADD, my heart is burned out. Can I rekindle my love for my husband?

Unfortunately, that's a little hard to tell. In my years of counseling, I've seen fairly cool ashes rekindled. I've also seen people who chose to go their separate ways and were glad they did so.

You need to get rather philosophical about this. If it's meant to be, it will be. In the meantime, don't try to force anything. Pressure is the kiss of death. Check with yourself to see how hard it feels to maintain the relationship. Look at little things to enjoy in each other and see what happens. Be open to feeling the sweetness of love. It can happen.

My wife left me because of my irresponsibility. Now, I believe I am ADD. Our marriage never had a chance. How do I get over feeling awful about what happened?

Attend to the grieving over the loss. Then find out all you can about ADD. Join a support group and start a new life for yourself. Learn from this day forward to make the most of what you have at any given moment. And learn from your experience so you don't make the same mistakes again.

Why don't people with ADD like surprises?

Surprises are intrusive. Though not all ADD people dislike surprises, sensitive people generally are going to feel the intrusion in extra measure. They also interrupt the steady flow of regularity. Remember, many people with ADD feel better and do better when they can count on what is going to happen.

If there is an emergency, what is the best way to get a person with ADD to react quickly?

Act as calmly as you can. In a very matter-of-fact way, convey the information about the emergency directly to the person from close range in a moderate to low voice. Try not to yell across the room. Measure your words, telling the person what you need for him or her to do.

Asking someone who's ADD to help you rather than giving direction is much more helpful in a crisis. Most people with ADD also like to know why they are being asked to do something: "I need you to immediately leave the house because it is on fire. If you will close the closet door, I will shut the kitchen door and meet you in the front yard."

INTIMATE RELATIONSHIPS

Achieving and maintaining an intimate relationship, both emotionally and physically, can be quite a challenge for both the

ADD person and the significant other. But, with an understanding of the ground rules—what works and what doesn't work—the return on the investment of your effort is highly rewarding.

As a couple, learn to manage your emotional balance. When you do, you can expect an easier road physically. It's pretty hard to have good physical relations with someone you don't respect or who is acting like your parent. So first of all, be sure to get your daily living under control so you each pull your own weight at home and outside the home. This means dividing up the responsibilities for moneymaking, child care, home maintenance, decision making, and a host of other things.

Each of you will be better at some things than at others. First, take responsibility for what each of you likes to do and does naturally. Next, divide up responsibility for what neither of you likes to do. This doesn't necessarily mean you personally do the job. It means you see that the job gets done, whether you do it yourself, make a trade with a friend to get it done, or pay to have it done. Naturally, you must consider your budget when you hire out, and you probably need to make that a joint activity.

Watch out for *flooding*. This is what happens when too much information or stimulation hits one of us ADD-style folks in a short time. As a partner to one of us who's flooded, you can help by gently questioning what's going on. Use a non-accusatory voice. If you slow your speech down a bit and soften your voice, you'll help soothe the frazzled nerves and mental chaos so that we can begin to think for ourselves again.

One ADD person I know admits to the following response to flooding: "When I'm flooded with information, I'm thinking of so many options that I can't do anything except yell, stomp off, or shut down. When this happens, what usually works is for my mate to say, 'What are you feeling right now? Tell me what you're thinking and we can go through the options one by one.' This kind of approach helps me focus on what I really want to do instead of being bombarded by a thousand other things."

Being able to tell your partner that a task is "just too hard" actually helps more sensitive intimacy develop between the two of you. Once you've said, "This is too hard for me because of my ADD," your partner comes to realize some of your limits and can sensitively respond. Such sensitivity is what intimacy is all about—the dance of understanding between two people when they are vulnerable, mutually dependent, and in need of trust from one another.

Both partners will find new levels of safety and feel appreciated and accepted. You'll be able to shift gears and share secrets, telling each other intimate and personal thoughts, and each of you will be able to ask for help without feeling vulnerable or overly dependent on the other.

Touching

Touching and being touched is tricky when two people have differences in their emotional and physical sensitivity. If you're ADD and stressed, you may not want to be touched at all until you decompress. It causes pain. But how do you tell someone you're close to that you can't handle being touched right now, without hurting his or her feelings?

When the partner needs or wants the contact, what can the person with ADD do that won't upset his partner but instead will convey a feeling of caring? One option to start with is the direct approach, followed by saying what you *can* manage: "I'm feeling very sensitive right now. Could I just hold your hand or give you a quick hug, or just sit next to you? That way I'll be able to relax with you soon. Then we can play." (Smile)

One woman wouldn't hug a man who had no awareness of his own strength. He always hurt her, even though she had told him many times that he was hurting her. His hugging felt painful. He just couldn't appreciate her sensitivity. So she ducked his hugs and smiled a lot.

Through small nuances and nonverbal communication, an ADD person often senses the ulterior motives of the person doing the hugging. In intimate relationships, sex may be on one partner's mind. But if that person starts out showing you sympathy and affection because you've had a hard day, you are likely, if you have an ADD brainstyle, to sense what is behind his approaching you. Generally, this kind of covert behavior breeds anger and rejection.

Rhythmic touch, such as repetitive stroking or patting, frequently annoys an ADD person. Instead, try gently and firmly taking an arm or a toe or one finger and hold it firmly. Although massage—the full-body type—may help reduce tension in many people, it may be just too much of a good thing to some. If you and your partner want to try massage as a pleasure-giving intimacy, try using oils to create a nonirritating touch, and keep the massage short, maybe 15–20 minutes.

Experiment with variations. Once something pleasant is discovered, there is a strong possibility that the ADD person will not want to stick with it for very long. In turn, the ADD person may find it difficult to believe that the non-ADD person likes the same thing repeatedly. Partners of ADD persons often find this phenomenon frustrating and have trouble getting the ADD person to repeat pleasurable touching.

Other tips: Try hugging from behind instead of from the front. Or try putting the head of the ADD person in your lap. But be careful when you put your arm over the shoulder of an ADD person, especially a woman. The weight may feel too heavy.

Sex

Sex—so individual that it's difficult to generalize about it without making people uncomfortable, without leaving someone out, or without violating someone's right to be different. Nevertheless, in relation to ADD people, there are some generalities I can outline.

The big generality is, simply, sex between an ADD person and another person requires understanding, or it's destined to cause frustration and dissatisfaction. This means that the ability to communicate verbally is essential to let personal needs and wants be known. It also takes understanding in reverse from the ADD person for the partner who may not want to do a lot of talking. Gently work your way to a middle ground with the understanding that there is no one right way, that each of you is different, and that in your love, you wish to bridge the differences.

From foreplay to location, variety is often the key to successful sex with an ADD person. Remember that boredom with the same thing (repetition) is one of the most frustrating, stress-producing feelings a person with ADD attributes has to deal with. Fortunately, at least for the ADD person, there's usually a willingness to experiment.

Vary the location and environment for sex. Don't just have it in the bedroom, but try the living room or backseat of the car. Try it in the swimming pool or shower. Try turning off the air conditioner in summer to build up a sweat. Switch from cotton sheets to satin sheets in the summer and flannel sheets in the winter. Remember, variety is the key for most ADD adults.

Creative sexual behavior is often pleasing. It does take a lot of trust and feelings of safety with the other person to be willing to go this route. And, if you are the one who wants to experiment and your partner is more reserved, you will have to reign in your creativity to let your partner catch up with you. What feels so, so good to a creative pleasurer may feel equally bad to someone who likes the security and comfort of sameness. Neither way is wrong or pathological. People are just different.

An ADD person can get a lot out of foreplay if the individuals are comfortable with sex and if they mutually like each other and want each other physically. Because of the tension-relieving nature of sex, foreplay often acts as a reminder of pleasures to come. And usually, there's not a problem concentrating on it, providing you keep it varied and it's not prolonged. This is true even when the relationship is full of fighting and conflict. Sex makes people feel that they have some control: "Here's a person I care about, and I have a guaranteed outcome."

If you are not in tune with your partner, loving and liking each other, the guaranteed outcome will probably be elusive. A person with ADD can then be rejecting, feeling intruded upon by the partner's sexual desires or blaming the partner for the problems they are having. It's important that the partner accepts no more than half the responsibility for the lack of fulfillment.

But, even with loving, caring couples, it's important to remember that ADD people are extremely sensitive to pleasure and pain and act accordingly. Sensitivity can be used to advantage, however. If you do it right, it leads to the greatest pleasure two people can share.

Some practical tips: One ADD person I know likes the light touch of fingernails drawn across her skin, but not too much in one place. Another likes being stroked with an ice cube, and still another likes being licked (try honey or chocolate)—but, again, never too long in one place.

Variation in sexual position follows the same rule of thumb: anything goes that will keep interest heightened for the creative, big-picture ADD person. Obviously, variation must be acceptable to both partners, not pursued at the expense of one. Oral sex can fill the need for diversity, but it is imperative that good hygiene be followed. Remember, all of the senses of a person with ADD are heightened. If his or her sense of smell or taste is offended, the desire for intimacy is squelched.

Because of the ADD person's sensitivity to pain, men must be especially mindful of finding comfortable positions for intercourse with an ADD female. And a female partner must not be offended or feel that she is unattractive because her ADD partner says, "You're too heavy." You can be perfectly average weight and be experienced as heavy by a sensitive person. It's not you. It's the other's sensitivity.

Good communication and willingness to be flexible are essential here. ADD persons of either sex will generally experience the pressure of weight on top of them as less comfortable than will non-ADD folks, so they may resist having the partner on top during intercourse. The key is understanding and the willingness to find positions that feel good to both participants.

Sexual Repression

There are exceptions, however, to these guidelines. After all, comfort with experimentation depends on how a person was trained about sex and whether he or she was raised with a sense of safety about it. Without such an upbringing, an ADD person may want no variability. Experimentation and prolonged sexual expression may seem too dangerous. Having sex the same way all the time may make him or her feel safe. Otherwise, he or she will make every effort to avoid sex—and exhibit rigidity. There will be a tendency to make sex mechanical.

When You're the Partner

Yes, there's a lot you can do for your partner with ADD characteristics, but let's not leave you out of the mix. It doesn't hurt to satisfy your mate's special needs, but yours need to be met, too. It's imperative that both participants are satisfied, no matter what their brainstyle: no losers. Communication and consensus are the keys to making this happen.

There's nothing wrong with saying, "It's my turn now." One day, do it her way, the next try it yours. Let your partner know what you like, and ask for it. Don't demand, whine, or scold. No one likes these approaches, and folks with ADD attributes are no different. They do, however, usually like humor, so it may do you well to add some instead of taking the sex game too seriously. Teasingly, you might say, "Watch out! I'll get you when you're least expecting it . . . okay, not really. But, let's play, huh?" It will be the lighthearted tone in your voice that will entice your lover.

Remember, the vulnerable feelings of an ADD person are soothed by reassurances that you won't hurt her. Better you learn to back off for a while than ruin the whole thing by impatiently trying to force sex. Say, "I'll stop if you want me to, but will you bring me to a climax?" It's important that the ADD person not leave you hanging, so communicate your needs.

Consensus, not compromise, is a couple's best friend. In consensus, together you find an alternative that pleases both of you. Don't give in and set yourself up as a loser. Don't act on feelings of impatience because you are having trouble finding the solution. Say, "I know we'll find what is good for both of us. I love you."

If your partner will not work with you, you may need to become very clear that you can't do it all yourself. Sex is one area in which you cannot succeed alone, and going outside the partnership for sexual gratification is questionable. It's better to face the fact that your partner is unwilling to work with you on sexual issues and get on with your life. Seek marriage counseling and be willing to call it quits if the willingness to try has vanished.

It is important to distinguish between a willingness to try and an ability to succeed. If you hear, "I'm sorry," then you at least know you are being considered. You may expect to be told you are important and lovable, which means your partner is taking responsibility for his part in this. ADD or not, no partner gets a free ride. Understanding? Yes! A free ride? No!

Trouble in relation to sex rarely is the cause of a troubled partnership. Rather it is the symptom of other problems with trust, control, respect, and thoughtfulness. Counseling may be needed to determine if your relationship can survive.

Brainstyle differences, properly respected and worked with, can enhance relationships tremendously. It's all a matter of appreciating differences and learning to enjoy them. They are truly more of an asset than a liability.

What was that phrase? Variety is the spice of life. ADD definitely can add spice to any relationship you're a part of. Enjoy yourself.

COMMON QUESTIONS ABOUT INTIMACY

My wife has trouble maintaining eye contact in a conversation with me, keeps fiddling with things, and gets up and moves around instead of paying attention to me. Is she bored with me, or could her behavior be caused by ADD?

What you're seeing might be due to her ADD brainstyle, and it might not be.

In an intimate relationship, ADD or not, you need to work at good communication. Ask your wife how she is feeling. Ask her whether it would be easier for her to talk with you if you are walking together.

Ask if it would help for you to talk in short segments. Maybe you belabor points, talking too long or in too much depth about simple matters. Check to see what the style of your conversation is. Do you lecture, scold, go on and on, talk down to her, talk only about yourself, or monopolize the conversation?

I feel hurt because of her behavior. What can I do to feel better?

Feeling hurt by the other person is a great way to wreck a relationship. It puts responsibility for how you feel on the other person. Sounds like something you learned from your own past.

To remedy the situation, do two basic things:

- Look at your own expectations to see what it is you think your wife ought to be doing for you. Then do it yourself.
- Ask your wife whether she intended to hurt you with her behavior. She'll probably look utterly amazed and say "No." Then adjust your thinking to reflect what you've learned.

My husband, who has an ADD brainstyle, might be called the one-minute lover. I'm not making fun of him; it's just true. He has no need for foreplay, especially anything I might need or prefer. I need more—more intimacy, more of everything. What can I do?

This discussion assumes that your spouse does not use alcohol to excess. Find a neutral time, not when you're already in bed, to talk about the situation. Start with something positive, such as how much you care about him and would like making love with him.

Determine whether he has gotten into a bad habit of being thoughtless about you or whether he is truly suffering from a condition called premature ejaculation. A marriage counselor, physician, or sex therapist can help you with the latter.

You and he can do a lot about the thoughtlessness. Ask for his help. Take small steps, asking for a little fondling at first. Tell him how important it is to you. Be careful not to blame, criticize, or scold him about his lovemaking. But do make your point that you are important and want to have fun, too.

Do not necessarily expect to climax at the same time as your husband. If he has already come, ask him to continue to make love to you until you do, too. Or turn it around and ask him to make love to you first.

Above all, do not make the remediation of the problem too serious. Add some fun along with a full measure of sensitivity, and enjoy one another. If, however, your husband persists in not paying heed to your needs, you may have to look deeper into the quality of your overall relationship with him. Then assess what you want out of a relationship.

Thoughtlessness is not due to an ADD style of brain construction.

I'm a hugger, toucher, and feeler. It's just the way I am. I'm married to an ADD person who really doesn't like to be touched, at least not in the way I like to touch. What can we do? How can one of us not lose in this situation? Are we doomed for frustration or divorce?

Since you are the one who likes to be touched, let her touch you rather than vice versa. I also wonder if you haven't been touching her as a way to initiate sex, which turns her off. Be clear about what you want, and you may have a deal.

The real trick in intimacy is to have no losers. There is always a loser if coercion is used. Therefore, you two must find ways to be together that satisfy both of you. To accomplish this, talk, experiment, and try some soothing oils. Be sure with your ADD wife that you touch her gently and firmly and don't stay in one place very long. No tickling unless she wants it.

I have ADD, and it takes me a long time to reach orgasm. I keep getting distracted, and my partner eventually gets bored. What's the solution?

Taking a long time to reach orgasm may not be the result of ADD. Neither is your distractibility. First, get a physical with a doctor you trust. Then, if all is okay, look for causative factors in what you were taught about sex and what your previous sexual experiences may have been.

If you were mistreated or were sexually abused, you would have learned to distract yourself as a psychological protection. It's hard to turn your awareness back on, even though it's now safe. Counseling offers a lot of good help for this kind of problem.

Finally, check to be sure you are attracted to your partner.

When I sleep, I like to be tucked under the covers and hold my wife like a pillow. She hates it and says it feels like she's being suffocated. Yet I have a hard time falling asleep without it. What can I do?

Better get yourself a real pillow to hug.

Occasionally embracing your wife would probably feel good to her. But, using her like a pillow for comfort is asking too much. Slowly wean yourself away from the habit.

My wife, who is ADD, is really adamant when she talks about what she likes sexually. Yet it seems that what she likes changes constantly. I get confused. What does she really like?

Variation.

In intimate relationships, ADD is only one of many factors that affect togetherness in all its forms. Good communication, thoughtful caring, willingness to give and take, and genuine love for your mate are required if your relationship is to blossom and endure. Forgiveness for differences is absolutely necessary. And willingness to walk in the other's path with empathy and understanding will go a long way to building a lasting relationship that you both can treasure.

EPILOGUE

Seven years ago, I wrote, "People who are ADD have been drawn to me like bears to honey. I, in turn, love the wonderful characteristics that are part of some of the sweetest, most sensitive people in the world. My personal friends are disproportionately weighted in that direction. The people I have connected with through radio, television, and public appearances frequently have had more than their fair share of ADD attributes, and my private practice brought me in touch with many others with whom I am able to work effectively. And, I have discovered that I am ADD."

Today, as I write the fourth edition, I have become aware of a number of changes in myself. I no longer seem to attract so many people with lots of ADD attributes—I attract some, but no more than people with a few or hardly any. My personal friends break down about equally between "lots," "some," and "few" attributes.

Even more astonishing is that my colleagues are rarely ADD. Part of this is because I'm doing more teamwork, and I *need* people who have skills different from my own. In retrospect, I didn't do teamwork in the early '90s. Now I do. Finally, though I'm still loaded with ADD attributes, they don't seem to be an issue, which is interesting because I no longer have a staff (other than an accountant) to do the jobs I don't naturally do well. I've just sort of found ways to get the things done that once were so very hard. Though I'm as ADD as ever, I seem more balanced—I'm not sure if that makes sense according to linear logic, but it makes sense to me.

In the past, I wondered why the magnetism between me and so many ADD persons had existed. I wrote, "The answer, I believe, lies in characteristics we share." I continued, saying, "I am very sensitive and feel things deeply. I am creative by nature and in my approach to problems." I mentioned being learning disabled as an explanation for knowing the feelings of lost potential firsthand.

I said, "I'm empathetic with regard to the feelings of others. I get bored easily, can't sit still, and don't organize (organize details) well—at least as judged by most people. All these traits I share with people who have an ADD brain wiring."

Ironically, I still have a magnetism of sorts to the people to whom I'm attracted. I am not casual about the people I spend a lot of time with. Actually, I'm very choosy, more than I used to be. Now, I believe the question of why I'm drawn to who I'm drawn to has a different answer. It's because they *are different* from me. They bring something I don't have.

I'm still the same sensitive, deeply feeling person I was before. I'm still creative and actually express my creativity much more than previously. I'm still learning disabled. But I no longer relate personally to the feeling of lost potential. Instead, I recall that I used to experience the feelings of lost potential firsthand. Then and now, I've been empathetic with regard to the feelings of others, but that too has changed. I know now that, both inwardly with emotions and outwardly with skill building, feelings can be transformed from something hurtful or challenging to the building blocks for understanding and accomplishment.

I still get bored easily, but seem to have so much that I truly *want* to do that I rarely feel bored. I basically don't do much of anything I don't want to do. How did I get to this point? By finally learning to be selective about how I spend my time and being aware of when something begins to get "boring," I begin the process of moving on—with a combination of searching and responsibility.

I'm much less impulsive than I once was, and I'm more patient, willing to wait for the right time and circumstances before I make my moves. I attribute this to the trust I've learned by healing my Wounded Self, learning to use my Accommodating Self, and freeing my True Self. I have faith that the natural way that my brain is constructed will serve me admirably to be who I was always meant to be.

As I look at what I've written, I'm reminded how children initially play alone or near others before they learn to play *with* others. Perhaps the changes I've experienced are simply due to normal growth and development. Perhaps it takes time for our natural talents and skills to mature, and only when they do can we use them effectively and effortlessly, without serious thought and intent. I've learned to use my ADD to my advantage.

Though I still admire the characteristics displayed by those of us who are ADD, I now realize how essential they are to the accomplishment of any job. They are needed to maintain biodiversity at all levels. Without well-developed ADD characteristics, the workplace and beyond will become increasingly off balance.

As I said in earlier editions as well as this one, the first step must be to heal the hurt that lack of understanding of brain diversity has wrought for us. But that is no longer enough. My attention is now increasingly focused on supporting individuals with ADD attributes, on embracing and developing them and seeing that a place is made for them in the marketplace of living.

To provide this support, I wish to begin by looking at some of my favorite advantages that ADD offers.

- It's difficult to fool people with ADD. We look past surface appearances and façades to the core of people and issues and evaluate them with down-to-earth standards. We may see the truth even when another person is unaware of it within himself.
    - The biggest problem with this ability comes from not believing in ourselves.
- We tend to be good networkers, because we see so many relationships between people and things.
    - The biggest problem with this ability is that we sometimes try to force an outcome instead of making the connection and then letting it take on a life of its own.
- Because we don't suffer from "boundary isolation," that is, separation from others because of strong boundaries around

ourselves with little awareness of what's beyond those boundaries (also called "focus"), we are able to put new projects together readily. (This is our creativity working for us.)

We can cross disciplines or skill areas, drawing from what attracts our attention. Without the boundaries that confine non-ADD people, we focus on relationships between things. Because we can so easily switch our attention from one thing to another, we don't get in a rut.

- We do need to develop the skills to stick with the projects and relationships made available to us. This takes belief that what we are doing is important and that the way in which we go about accomplishing our goal is just fine.

- People with lots of ADD attributes tend to be "original" in both thought and the way in which we move from one thing to another. Our zigzag lines of pursuit serve us well if we let them. We don't miss a cue. At the best of times, we are fun to go places with because we see things other people don't see. We are truly creative.

    - Living creatively may not be the easiest path to follow for anyone in this culture. But those who believe in their creativity and really cannot live any other way can be very happy.

Misunderstood as you may be, you must know that you are one of the great unrecognized treasures of our land. You are a natural resource that can be tapped. Additional support to make use of ADD gifts will take understanding, adjustments in the educational process to better fit our style of learning, improved assessment of our skills, and awareness on the part of parents so that they can adjust their parenting styles to avoid the hurt and damage to the next generation of adults.

Our biggest hurdle will be to learn to trust ourselves so we can show future generations how valuable the ADD way is. Children and adults alike must find models who they can emulate and who can help teach them to adjust the functioning of their brainstyle to fit into a culture that, to date, hasn't favored it.

With this kind of teaching, children and adults will be able to speak out about brain diversity. They will be able to become teammates in work and learning environments so they, as all workers and learners, can use their talents and gifts effectively.

APPENDIX

APPENDIX A

NEW ADD ASSESSMENT CHECKLIST

Answer the following questions about yourself. If you've spent time learning to accommodate the situation or feeling, reference your answer to a time before you did your self work.

You may also find it helpful to have someone else answer these questions in relation to you.

	Yes	Some	No
Do you often fail to finish detailed tasks?	____	____	____
Do you have trouble managing your checkbook and finances?	____	____	____
Are you easily distracted when dealing with details, paperwork, and administrative tasks?	____	____	____
Do you get bored doing repetitive tasks?	____	____	____
Do you get bored or lose attention with sustained-action tasks?	____	____	____

	Yes	Some	No
Do you rarely do careful long-term planning even with major decisions?	____	____	____
Have you teamed up with people who manage details and organize for you?	____	____	____
Do you feel you've achieved below your potential in school or at work?	____	____	____
Do you frequently act without thinking?	____	____	____
Do you multitask, doing more than one thing at a time?	____	____	____
Do you work better when shifting from one activity to another?	____	____	____
Do you stick with one task until it is done?	____	____	____
Do you have many interests that you enjoy for a while, then drop regardless of financial investment?	____	____	____
Have you struggled with substance abuse?	____	____	____
Do you respond better to being asked than being told?	____	____	____
Do you have a sense of humor?	____	____	____
Do your eyes twinkle?	____	____	____
Do you call and talk out, interrupting conversations?	____	____	____
Do you get restless waiting your turn in a group situation?	____	____	____
Do you feel impatient or express your impatience with boring or slow-moving situations?	____	____	____
Is it hard for you to structure your environment?	____	____	____

	Yes	Some	No
Does your creativity feel cramped by too much structure?	____	____	____
Do you often finish another's sentences?	____	____	____
Do you prefer activity over stillness most of the time?	____	____	____
Do you become sleepy or restless if not active?	____	____	____
Is it hard for you to sit still?	____	____	____
Is it hard for you to stay seated?	____	____	____
Have you frequently changed jobs regardless of the reason?	____	____	____
Do you think better when you're active?	____	____	____
Have you often had periods of depression?	____	____	____
Are you very sensitive emotionally?	____	____	____
Do you take things personally or get your feelings hurt easily?	____	____	____
Are you very sensitive to hidden agendas or do you know what others are feeling even if they try to hide it?	____	____	____
Do you have a wide range of emotions?	____	____	____
Does your mood shift dramatically based on the people and events around you?	____	____	____
Do you have a quick temper that also disappears quickly when the situation is no longer threatening?	____	____	____
Are you physically sensitive to people or things?	____	____	____
Are you soothed and/or aided in focusing by the use of a TV, radio, or fan?	____	____	____

	Yes	Some	No
Are you empathetic?	____	____	____
Do you have trouble getting places on time?	____	____	____
Do you have difficulty determining how long a task will take?	____	____	____

APPENDIX B

DSM-IV DEFINITION OF ADD/ADHD: OFFICIAL DIAGNOSIS OF ADD IN ADULTS

AMERICAN PSYCHIATRIC ASSOCIATION *DIAGNOSTIC AND STATISTICAL MANUAL (DSM-IV)*

The fourth edition of the *APA Diagnostic and Statistical Manual* was published in 1994. Though not fully revised, the *DSM-IV-TR* was released with modifications in 2000. In it, the category for Attention Deficit/Hyperactivity Disorder (ADHD) was unchanged. ADD is listed in a section entitled "Usually First Diagnosed in Infancy, Childhood or Adolescence." According to the manual, diagnosis can be made with either of two sets of symptoms. The first focuses on *inattention.*

According to the *DSM-IV*, for an adult to be diagnosed with ADD, he or she must have had problems in six of the following areas for at least six months.

A. Fails to give close attention to details.

B. Has difficulty sustaining attention.

C. Often doesn't seem to listen.

D. Experiences problems with follow-through or finishing work.

E. Has difficulty organizing tasks and activities.

F. Frequently avoids and dislikes sustained-action tasks.

G. Loses things needed for tasks.

H. Is easily distracted by extraneous stimuli.

I. Is forgetful in daily activities.

The second set of symptoms focuses on *hyperactivity/impulsivity* and also requires six symptoms persisting for six months.

A. Fidgets with hands or feet or squirms in seat.

B. Leaves seat when expected to remain seated.

C. Experiences feelings of restlessness.

D. Has trouble engaging in leisure activities quietly.

E. Is "on the go" often or "driven by a motor."

F. Talks excessively.

G. Blurts out answers before question is complete.

H. Has difficulty awaiting turn.

I. Interrupts or intrudes on others.

The behaviors must be present before age seven; they must be present in two or more settings, such as school, work, or home; and the impairment must be visible in social, academic, or occupational settings.

Three subtypes are noted in the *DSM-IV*. Each has a diagnostic code that must be used when dealing with insurance companies and other official agencies. The manual states that most individuals have symptoms of both inattention and hyperactivity/impulsivity. Often, however, one or the other pattern is predominant. For a current adult diagnosis, one of the subtypes needs to be noted.

314.00 Attention Deficit/Hyperactivity Disorder, Predominantly Inattentive Type. This subtype should be used if six (or more) symptoms of inattention (but fewer than six symptoms of hyperactivity/impulsivity) have persisted for at least six months.

314.01 Attention Deficit/Hyperactivity Disorder, Combined Type. This subtype should be used if six (or more) symptoms of inattention and six (or more) symptoms of hyperactivity/impulsivity have persisted for at least six months. Most children and adolescents with the disorder have the Combined Type. It is not known whether the same is true of adults with the disorder.

314.01 Attention Deficit/Hyperactivity Disorder, Predominantly Hyperactive/Impulsive Type. This subtype should be used if six (or more) symptoms of hyperactivity but fewer than six symptoms of inattention have persisted for at least six months. Inattention may often still be a significant feature in such cases.

Future revisions of the *Diagnostic and Statistical Manual* are likely to further modify these criteria.

APPENDIX C

RESEARCH BIBLIOGRAPHY

Barkley, R. A. (1997). *ADHD and the Nature of Self-Control.* New York: Guilford.

Barkley, R. A. (1998). *Attention-Deficit Hyperactivity Disorder: A Handbook for Diagnosis and Treatment* (2nd edition). New York: Guilford.

Baumeister, A., & Hawkins, M. (2001). Incoherence of Neuro-imaging Studies of Attention Deficit/Hyperactivity Disorder. *Clinical Neuro-Pharmacology, 24* (1), 2–10.

Biederman, J., Faraone, S. V., Mick, E., Spencer, T., Wilens, T., Kiely, K., Guite, J., Ablun, J. S., Reed, E., & Warburton, R. (1995). High Risk for Attention Deficit Hyperactivity Disorder among Children of Parents with Childhood Onset of the Disorder. *American Journal of Psychiatry, 152*, 431–435.

Cloniger, R. C., Surakic, D. M., & Przyback, T. R. (1993). A Psychological Model of Temperament and Character. *Archives of General Psychiatry, 50*, 973–990.

Durston, S., Hulshoff Pol, H. E., Casey, B. J., Giudd, R. N., Buitelaar, J. D., and van Engeland, H. (2001). Anatomical MRI of the Developing Human Brain: What Have We Learned? *Journal of the American Academy of Child and Adolescent Psychiatry, 40* (9), 1012–1020.

Faraone, S. V. (2000). Genetics of Childhood Disorders: XIX. ADHD, Part 4: Is ADHD Genetically Heterogeneous? *Journal of American Academy of Child and Adolescent Psychiatry, 39* (11), 1201–1205.

Fernandez-Duque, D., & Posner, M. I. (2001). Brain Imaging of Attentional Networks in Normal and Pathological States. *Journal of Clinical and Experimental Neuropsychology, 23* (1), 74–93.

Frank, Y., & Pavlakis, S. G. (2001). Brain Imaging in Neurobehavioral Disorders. *Pediatric Neurology, 25* (4), 278–287.

Galves, A. O., Cohen, D., Dunlap, M., Greening, T., Karon, B. P., Simon, L., et al. (2004). Personal communication, April 29.

Kuhn, T. (1962). *The Structure of Scientific Revolutions*. Chicago: University of Chicago Press.

Kuo, F. E., & Faber Taylor, A. (2004). A Potential Natural Treatment for ADHD: Evidence from a National Study. *American Journal of Public Health, 94,* 1580–1586.

Leo, J. T., & Cohen, D. (2002). Broken Brains or Flawed Studies? A Critical Review of ADHD Neuro-imaging Research. *Journal of Mind and Behavior, 24,* 29–56.

Murray, B. (2003). Training Young Minds Not to Wander. *Monitor on Psychology* (October), 58–59.

Ochsner, K. N., & Lieberman, M. D. (2001). The Emergence of Social Cognitive Neuroscience. *American Psychologist, 56* (9), 717–734.

Overmeyer, S., & Taylor, E. (2001). Neuro-imaging in Hyperkinetic Children and Adults: An Overview. *Pediatric Rehabilitation, 4* (2), 57–70.

Stern, E., & Silbersweig, D. A. (2001). Advances in Functional Neuroimaging Methodology for the Study of Brain Systems Underlying Human Neuropsychological Function and Dysfunction. *Journal of Clinical and Experimental Neuropsychology, 12* (1), 3–18.

Sternberg, R. J., & Grisorenko, E. L. (1997). Are Cognitive Styles Still in Style? *American Psychologist, 51* (7), 700–712.

Tyron, W. W. (2002). Network Models Contribute to Cognitive and Social Neuroscience. *American Psychologist, 57* (9), 728.

Westen, D., & Weinberger, J. (2004). When Clinical Description Becomes Statistical Prediction. *American Psychologist, 59* (7), 595–613.

APPENDIX D

MEDICATION LIST AND TABLE

Keith Caramelli, M.D.

Ritalin: Manufactured by Novartis (formerly Ciba Geigy); generic is methylphenidate. A stimulant with side effects shared by all stimulants, including appetite suppression, insomnia, upset stomach, and occasional nervousness. All stimulants are controlled substances because they can be habituating. Onset of action is approximately one hour; duration of action is three to four hours. All stimulants have similar positive effects, improving focus, decreasing distractibility, and decreasing excess psychomotor activity. Pharmacological action is primarily through the actions of the neurotransmitter dopamine.

Focalin: Manufactured by Celgene, aka Novartis; generic is d-methylphenidate. Chemical compounds such as methylphenidate may have two forms or shapes, known as "isomers." With methylphenidate, it was felt that one of these "isomers" could be eliminated, resulting in the removal of many of the side effects without sacrificing any of the therapeutic action. While it is unclear how much the side-effect profile has been improved, it does appear that Focalin may last one to two hours longer than Ritalin (regular methylphenidate).

Adderall: For adults, manufactured by Shire US; for children, manufactured by Richwood Pharmaceutical Co.; generic is amphetamine sulphate. A stimulant with side effects shared by all stimulants. More potent per milligram than Ritalin, it shares the attributes and actions of Ritalin. Adderall may be more likely to cause the side effects shared by all stimulants. Pharmacological action is primarily through the actions of the neurotransmitters norepinephrine and dopamine.

Dexedrine: Manufactured by GlaxoSmithKline; generic is dextroamphetamine. A stimulant with side effects shared by all stimulants. Although a long-acting form has been available for quite a while (Dexedrine spansules), its efficacy has been less than satisfactory, and the other stimulants have since come out with more effective long-acting versions of their medicine, leaving Dexedrine rarely used these days.

Concerta: Manufactured by Alza; generic is methylphenidate. A long-acting form of methylphenidate that causes the gradual sustained release of the medicine from the capsule in the stomach. Onset of action may be slower (one hour), though duration of action may be up to 12 hours.

Ritalin LA: Manufactured by Novartis; generic is methylphenidate. A long-acting version of methylphenidate whose long action is accomplished by the active ingredient (methylphenidate) being encapsulated in multiple tiny beads within the capsule, half of the beads dissolving rapidly in the stomach and the other half dissolving after three to four hours, effectively giving a second burst of methylphenidate after the first half dissolves.

Metadate CD: Manufactured by Celltech Pharmaceuticals, Ltd.; generic is methylphenidate. A long-acting version of methylphenidate with a mechanism similar to Ritalin LA. Tolerated well by some when Ritalin LA is not and vice versa.

Table Appendix D.1

Medication	*Frequency*	*Peak Effect*	*Duration of Action*
Dexedrine (d-amphetamine)	2 or 3 times per day	1–3 hours	5 hours
Dexedrine spansules	Once in a.m.	2–3 hours	9 hours
Adderall	2 or 3 times per day	1–3 hours	5 hours
Adderall XR	Once in a.m.	1–4 hours	9 hours
Ritalin	3 times per day	1–3 hours	2–4 hours
Focalin	2 times per day	1–4 hours	2–5 hours
Ritalin LA	Once in a.m.	4–5 hours	8 hours
Metadate CD	Once in a.m.	5 hours	8 hours
Concerta	Once in a.m.	8 hours	12 hours

Adderall XR: Manufactured by Shire (adults) and Richwood Pharmaceutical Co. (children); generic is amphetamine sulphate. A long-acting version of amphetamine sulphate whose long action is accomplished through a similar mechanism to Ritalin LA and Metadate CD. The active ingredient is encased in tiny beads, half of which dissolve quickly in the stomach and half of which dissolve after three to four hours, releasing the second dose of Adderall into the body.

Cylert: Manufactured by Abbott; generic is pemoline. Some stimulant action, but not a stimulant in the traditional sense. A long-acting ADHD compound that has been available for some time though is traditionally less effective than the "stimulants." Since long-acting forms of the stimulants have become available and rare serious side effects have been found with Cylert (liver toxicity), it is infrequently used.

Strattera: Manufactured by Eli Lilly; generic is atomoxetine, a recently developed nonstimulant ADHD medication; attributes are largely an improvement in concentration and focus. Although impulsivity may be improved, the effects on hyperactivity are probably less than with the stimulants. Strattera is long acting, with a suspected duration of action greater than 24 hours. Unlike stimulants, Strattera does not have an onset of action on the day that it is taken and requires at least five days (if not up to 30) of continual administration to see it's therapeutic effects. Consequently, Strattera requires daily administration to be effective (in contrast to the stimulants) but also does not wear off in the evening, which may cause problems with the stimulant medications. Side effects include appetite suppression, nausea, sedation, and elevation of blood pressure. Strattera works on the neurotransmitter norepinephrine.

Welbutrin: Manufactured by GlaxoSmithKline; generic is buproprion. An antidepressant with some significant efficacy for improvement in concentration and focus. Actions on hyperactive behavior are few. Antidepressants require at least three to four weeks of daily administration to be effective. Side effects include milder appetite suppression than the above compounds, nervousness, insomnia, and a susceptibility to seizures in individuals with a history of epilepsy.

Effexor: Manufactured by Wyeth; generic is venlafaxine. An antidepressant with some efficacy on concentration and focus. Action on hyperactive behavior is little. Side effects include nausea, headache, dizziness, and elevation in blood pressure. Abrupt discontinuation of Effexor can create uncomfortable side effects.

APPENDIX E

AMERICANS WITH DISABILITIES ACT

The Americans with Disabilities Act (ADA) is designed to provide people with a "disability" fair chance to succeed at a job or in an educational setting for which they have the skills and abilities, but who need accommodation in order to show what they are able to do. For example, if a student knows the material being tested for, but cannot show that knowledge because of the style of the test being given, then accommodation might provide a means of testing that will demonstrate what the student knows.

People with ADD characteristics must not use ADA so that they can study subjects or stay in jobs that are not suited to their overall capability. It is also not meant to be the first step when problems arise at school or on the job. Often it is not necessary to wave an ADD flag in a teacher's or boss's face *demanding* changes and help. Rather, simply providing the person with information about how you can do your job or learn your schoolwork may yield accommodation without ever mentioning, much less threatening to invoke, the Americans with Disabilities Act.

The major drawback to ADA is that it requires you to say you're "disabled." In line with the theme of this book, equal opportunity legislation comes closer to the mark of what you require than ADA. You and others deserve an equal opportunity to show what you know because an ADD brainstyle is nothing more than a form of diversity—diversity of brainstyle. But because of the belief that people with an ADD brainstyle are defective or disordered, you are required to state you are disabled in order to be given the accommodation that is the birthright of all people.

If the time comes when you have exhausted other means to succeed in a situation that is demanded of you, but one that you are struggling with as a means to an end that fits your brainstyle, you may decide to enlist the Americans with Disabilities Act. As you do, simply keep in mind that there is actually nothing *wrong* with you. Remember that societal beliefs take time to change. Meanwhile, there is no reason your dreams should crash and burn. Instead call upon ADA.

The easiest way to gain information about the Americans with Disabilities Act is by going to the Web. You will find numerous sites of interest. Use a search engine such as Google and type in the following subject: "Americans with Disabilities + Attention Deficit Disorder" or "Americans with Disabilities + Attention Deficit Disorder + education." You will see lists of sites regarding the use of ADA in employment and ADA in school.

With thoughtful, responsible communication about the kinds of accommodation that will help you reach your goals, you may never need to legally use ADA. But should you decide to, remember it is a tool to help you do what fits the True You and remember that there is actually nothing *wrong* with you because you're taking this step.

The following material is taken from the Americans with Disabilities Act website that you can access most easily by doing a search: "Americans with Disabilities Act + Attention Deficit Disorder." Also see below for more specific information.

SOURCES OF INFORMATION ABOUT THE AMERICANS WITH DISABILITIES ACT

If you are thinking about filing a discrimination complaint under the ADA or would just like additional information about your rights, there are many sources of free information. Your public library is likely to have the latest information about the Americans with Disabilities Act. The government sent 95 ADA publications and a videotape about the ADA to 15,000 libraries across the country. Here are some other sources, which have been adapted from publications of the Disability Rights Section of the U.S. Department of Justice:

- **U.S. Equal Employment Opportunity Commission**

  1801 L Street, NW Washington, DC 20007

  800-669-4000 (to ask questions about employment or for help locating your local field office)

  800-669-3362 (to order documents)

  Web site: http://www.eeoc.gov

  The EEOC offers technical assistance on the ADA provisions applying to employment and also provides information on how to file ADA complaints.

- **The Disability Rights Education and Defense Fund** (DREDF) ADA Hotline 800-466-4232.

  This hotline is funded by the Department of Justice to provide technical assistance on the Americans with Disabilities Act. Call the hotline to ask questions or order publications about the ADA.

- **President's Committee on Employment of People with Disabilities**

  1331 F Street, NW Washington, DC 20004

  202-376-6200 (employment questions)

  Web site: http://www.dol.gov/odep/welcome.html

  The President's Committee answers employment questions and funds the Job Accommodation Network, below.

- **Job Accommodation Network**

  800-526-7234

  Web site: http://janweb.icdi.wvu.edu

  The network has a database of thousands of accommodations. Telephone consultants can provide personalized advice on accommodating employees with disabilities.

- **Center for Learning Disabilities and the Law**

  P.O. Box 368 Cabin John, MD 20818

  301-469-8308

> *The CLDL is a nonprofit organization that provides some counseling, but cannot return all calls. They are the only national organization that specializes in learning disabilities and the law.*

Be patient when you call these organizations. Some of the 800 numbers receive so many calls that you may have to hold or wait to have your call returned. And be ready with specific questions to ask. Do not try to tell your entire story on the telephone. Thank everyone who does a good job helping you.

CONCLUSION

The Americans with Disabilities Act can protect you against job discrimination from all except the smallest employers. Knowing your rights should give you confidence as you search for a job. Once you are offered a job, knowing your rights should also help you negotiate the accommodations you need.

APPENDIX F

RESOURCES

ADD-ON, INC.: ATTENTION DIVERSITY DISCOVERY ORGANIZATION

Attention Diversity Discovery Organization is a 501-3C non-profit organization that assisting individuals with an ADD style of brain construction in three ways:

1. It provides identification and education about ADD as a matter of diversity. Individuals will be able to find and utilize their True Selves to advantage.
2. It provides training and teaching of the skills that will help people accommodate to a society and environments that are not ADD-friendly so that wounding does not occur.
3. It assists in the healing of wounds that has resulted from misunderstanding and inappropriate handling of ADD individuals throughout their lives.

This fledgling organization is based on the philosophy forwarded in this book. Interested people are invited to contact the following website for more information.

www.theADD-Way.org

There are other resources available to people with an ADD brainstyle. However, the orientation reflected in most of the material, training, and conferences utilizes the medical model that starts with the premise that there is something wrong with a person with Attention Deficit Disorder.

Because this book takes the attitude that each of you must make choices with regard to the way in which you are constructed, I am including information for reaching two major organizations that have been active in work with ADD in adults. Each has over a decade of experience, and you will find many resources in relation to different aspects of ADD. Take what pleases you. And remember, there is nothing *wrong* with you.

ADDA
www.add.org
P.O. Box 543
Pottstown, PA 19464
(484) 945-2101

CHADD
www.chadd.org
8181 Professional Place, Ste. 150
Landover, MD 20785
(301) 306-7070
National Resource Center for AD/HD
(800) 233-4050

By doing an Internet search using the subject ADD/ADHD, you will find additional information.

OTHER TITLES PUBLISHED BY LYNN WEISS, PH.D.

The New ADD in Adults Workbook

View from the Cliff: A Course in Achieving Daily Focus

A.D.D. and Success

A.D.D. and Creativity

Give Your A.D.D. Teen a Chance

A.D.D. on the Job

The Attention Deficit Disorder in Adults Workbook

Attention Deficit Disorder in Adults:
Practical Help and Understanding

ABOUT THE AUTHOR

A psychotherapist for forty years, Lynn Weiss has an extensive backgroud in training, teaching, program development, and writing about human behavior and child development. For the past two decades, she's concentrated on forwarding an enlightened perspective on Attention Deficit Disorder as a brainstyle diversity issue.

Clinically trained through a NIMH clinical fellowship at the University of Washington Medical School, Dr. Weiss has brought her education to a practical level that builds from the health and strength in those with whom she comes in contact. She currently is writing non-fiction and fiction for adults and children and doing program development for natural resource managers as well as A.D.D. from her home in the woods in Central Texas.